Clinicians' Guides to Radionuclide Hybrid Imaging

PET/CT

W0050720

Series editors

Jamshed B. Bomanji
London, UK

Gopinath Gnanasegaran
London, UK

Stefano Fanti
Bologna, Italy

Homer A. Macapinlac
Houston, Texas, USA

More information about this series at http://www.springer.com/series/13803

Nilendu Purandare • Sneha Shah

Editors

PET/CT in Hepatobiliary and Pancreatic Malignancies

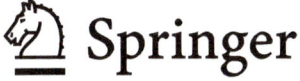 Springer

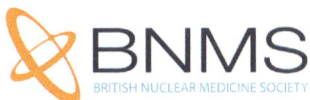

Editors
Nilendu Purandare
Department of Nuclear Medicine and
    Molecular Imaging
Tata Memorial Hospital
Mumbai
Maharashtra
India

Sneha Shah
Department of Nuclear Medicine and
    Molecular Imaging
Tata Memorial Hospital
Mumbai
Maharashtra
India

Clinicians' Guides to Radionuclide Hybrid Imaging - PET/CT
ISBN 978-3-319-60506-7   ISBN 978-3-319-60507-4   (eBook)
DOI 10.1007/978-3-319-60507-4

Library of Congress Control Number: 2017952346

Printed on acid-free paper

This Springer imprint is published by Springer Nature
The registered company is Springer International Publishing AG
The registered company address is: Gewerbestrasse 11, 6330 Cham, Switzerland

PET/CT series is dedicated to Prof. Ignac Fogelman, Dr. Muriel Buxton-Thomas and Prof. Ajit K. Padhy

Foreword

Clear and concise clinical indications for PET/CT in the management of the oncology patient are presented in this series of 15 separate booklets.

The impact on better staging, tailored management and specific treatment of the patient with cancer has been achieved with the advent of this multimodality imaging technology. Early and accurate diagnosis will always pay, and clear information can be gathered with PET/CT on treatment responses. Prognostic information is gathered and can guide additional therapeutic options.

It is a fortunate coincidence that PET/CT was able to derive great benefit from radionuclide-labelled probes, which deliver good and often excellent target to non-target signals. Whilst labelled glucose remains the cornerstone for the clinical benefit achieved, a number of recent probes are definitely adding benefit. PET/CT is hence an evolving technology, extending its applications and indications. Significant advances in the instrumentation and data processing available have also contributed to this technology, which delivers high throughput and a wealth of data, with good patient tolerance and indeed patient and public acceptance. As an example, the role of PET/CT in the evaluation of cardiac disease is also covered, with emphasis on labelled rubidium and labelled glucose studies.

The novel probes of labelled choline; labelled peptides, such as DOTATATE; and, most recently, labelled PSMA (prostate-specific membrane antigen) have gained rapid clinical utility and acceptance, as significant PET/CT tools for the management of neuroendocrine disease and prostate cancer patients, notwithstanding all the advances achieved with other imaging modalities, such as MRI. Hence, a chapter reviewing novel PET tracers forms part of this series.

The oncological community has recognised the value of PET/CT and has delivered advanced diagnostic criteria for some of the most important indications for PET/CT. This includes the recent Deauville criteria for the classification of PET/CT patients with lymphoma – similar criteria are expected to develop for other malignancies, such as head and neck cancer, melanoma and pelvic malignancies. For completion, a separate section covers the role of PET/CT in radiotherapy planning, discussing the indications for planning biological tumour volumes in relevant cancers.

These booklets offer simple, rapid and concise guidelines on the utility of PET/CT in a range of oncological indications. They also deliver a rapid aide-memoire on the merits and appropriate indications for PET/CT in oncology.

London, UK   Peter J. Ell, F.Med.Sci., DR HC, AΩA

Preface

Hybrid imaging with PET/CT and SPECT/CT combines best of function and structure to provide accurate localisation, characterisation and diagnosis. There is extensive literature and evidence to support PET/CT, which has made significant impact in oncological imaging and management of patients with cancer. The evidence in favour of SPECT/CT especially in orthopaedic indications is evolving and increasing.

The *Clinicians' Guides to Hybrid Imaging* (PET/CT and SPECT/CT) pocket book series is specifically aimed at our referring clinicians, nuclear medicine/radiology doctors, radiographers/technologists, and nurses who are routinely working in nuclear medicine and participate in multidisciplinary meetings. This series is the joint work of many friends and professionals from different nations who share a common dream and vision towards promoting and supporting nuclear medicine as a useful and important imaging speciality.

We want to thank all those people who have contributed to this work as advisors, authors and reviewers, without whom the book would not have been possible. We want to thank our members from the BNMS (British Nuclear Medicine Society, UK) for their encouragement and support, and we are extremely grateful to Dr. Brian Nielly, Charlotte Weston, the BNMS Education Committee and the BNMS Council members for their enthusiasm and trust.

Finally, we wish to extend particular gratitude to the industry for their continuous support towards education and training.

London, UK   Gopinath Gnanasegaran
                                                                                 Jamshed Bomanji

Acknowledgements

The series coordinators and editors would like to express sincere gratitude to the members of the British Nuclear Medicine Society, patients, teachers, colleagues, students, the industry and the BNMS Education Committee members, for their continued support and inspiration:

Andy Bradley
Brent Drake
Francis Sundram
James Ballinger
Parthiban Arumugam
Rizwan Syed
Sai Han
Vineet Prakash

Contents

Contributors

Archi Agrawal Department of Nuclear Medicine and Molecular Imaging, Tata Memorial Centre, Mumbai, Maharashtra, India

Kedar Deodhar Department of Pathology, Tata Memorial Hospital, Mumbai, Maharashtra, India

Ashwin deSouza Department of Gastrointestinal and HPB Surgery, Tata Memorial Centre, Mumbai, Maharashtra, India

Kunal Gala Department of Radiology, Tata Memorial Hospital, Mumbai, Maharashtra, India

Suyash Kulkarni Department of Radiology, Tata Memorial Hospital, Mumbai, Maharashtra, India

Ashwin Polnaya Department of Radiology, Tata Memorial Hospital, Mumbai, Maharashtra, India

Nilendu Purandare Department of Nuclear Medicine and Molecular Imaging, Tata Memorial Centre, Mumbai, Maharashtra, India

Ameya D. Puranik Department of Nuclear Medicine and Molecular Imaging, Tata Memorial Centre, Mumbai, Maharashtra, India

Venkatesh Rangarajan Department of Nuclear Medicine and Molecular Imaging, Tata Memorial Centre, Mumbai, Maharashtra, India

Sneha Shah Department of Nuclear Medicine and Molecular Imaging, Tata Memorial Centre, Mumbai, Maharashtra, India

Nitin Shetty Department of Radiology, Tata Memorial Hospital, Mumbai, Maharashtra, India

Hepatobiliary and Pancreatic Malignancies: Epidemiology, Clinical Presentation, Diagnosis, and Staging

Ashwin deSouza

Contents

1.1 Introduction

Hepatobiliary and pancreatic malignancies constitute a diverse range of disease processes, each with its own pathogenesis, presentation, and staging. This chapter will summarize the epidemiology, clinical presentation, diagnosis, and staging of hepatocellular carcinoma, carcinoma of the gall bladder and bile ducts, and pancreatic cancer.

A. deSouza, M.S., M.Ch., M.R.C.S.Ed., D.N.B.
Department of Gastrointestinal and HPB Surgery, Tata Memorial Centre,
Mumbai, Maharashtra, India
e-mail: ashwindesouza@gmail.com

1.2   Hepatocellular Carcinoma

1.2.1   Epidemiology and Etiology

Worldwide, hepatocellular carcinoma (HCC) is the fifth and seventh most common cancer in adult men and women, respectively. It also constitutes the second leading cause of cancer-related deaths in men and the sixth leading cause of cancer-related deaths in women [1].

In the majority of patients, HCC occurs in the setting of chronic liver disease. Nearly 80% of cases are due to underlying chronic hepatitis B and C infection [2] although cirrhosis of almost any cause is known to predispose to HCC.

Men are more likely to develop HCC as compared to women [1] with a mean age at presentation of 50–60 years [3, 4].

The various etiological factors of HCC are listed in Table 1.1.

1.2.2   Clinical Presentation

Patients with HCC usually present in advanced stages of the disease because of the absence of pathognomonic symptoms [5, 6]. The median survival following diagnosis is approximately 6–20 months [7].

Patients are largely asymptomatic, apart from symptoms of existing chronic liver disease. A diagnosis of HCC should be suspected in situations of recent onset hepatic decompensation in a patient with compensated chronic liver disease. Table 1.2 lists the common presenting symptoms and signs. Tumor rupture with intraperitoneal bleed is a rare clinical presentation which requires urgent resuscitation, angioembolization, or even surgery.

HCC can occasionally be associated with paraneoplastic syndromes like hypoglycemia, erythrocytosis, hypercalcemia, or severe watery diarrhea.

Table 1.1 Etiological/predisposing factors for hepatocellular carcinoma	
	Hepatitis B viral infection
	Chronic hepatitis C virus (HCV) infection
	Hereditary hemochromatosis
	Chronic hepatitis and cirrhosis
	Aflatoxin
	Contaminated drinking water
	Betel nut chewing
	Tobacco and alcohol abuse
	Diabetes mellitus
	Nonalcoholic fatty liver disease
	Obesity
	Iron overload
	Alpha-1 antitrypsin deficiency
	Acute intermittent porphyria
	Gallstones and cholecystectomy
	Dietary factors—consumption of red meat and saturated fat

Table 1.2 Hepatocellular carcinoma—clinical presentation

Symptoms
  - Asymptomatic—incidental finding
  - Jaundice, anorexia, weight loss, malaise
  - Vague upper abdominal pain
  - Upper abdominal mass
  - Acute presentation—intralesional bleed with acute onset severe abdominal pain, intraperitoneal rupture with bleed

Signs
  - Hepatomegaly (50–90%)
  - Hepatic bruit (6–25%)
  - Ascites (30–60%)
  - Splenomegaly due to associated portal hypertension from underlying liver disease
  - Fever (10–50%)—probably due to tumor necrosis
  - Signs of chronic liver disease—jaundice, dilated abdominal veins, palmar erythema, gynecomastia, testicular atrophy, and peripheral edema
  - Budd-Chiari syndrome due to invasion into the hepatic veins causes tense ascites and large tender liver
  - Troisier's sign—left supraclavicular lymph node enlargement (Virchow's node)

1.2.3   Diagnosis and Staging

Triple-phase contrast-enhanced CT scan or MRI is the investigative modality of choice for HCC. A diagnosis of HCC can be made for a solid liver lesion with characteristic enhancement patterns, i.e., enhancement in the arterial phase and contrast washout in the venous phase. Both arterial enhancement and venous washout are essential to make a diagnosis of HCC.

As the majority of patients with HCC have pre-existing chronic liver disease, enrolling these patients into a surveillance program of 6-monthly ultrasound aids in early diagnosis. Fig. 1.1 shows the American Association for the Study of Liver Diseases (AASLD) algorithm for suspected HCC [8]. Differentiation between high-grade dysplastic nodules and HCC on biopsy may be challenging and requires evaluation by expert pathologists supplemented with staining for glypican 3, heat shock protein 70, and glutamine synthetase. If the biopsy is negative for HCC, patients should be followed by imaging at 3- to 6-month intervals until the nodule either disappears, enlarges, or displays diagnostic characteristics of HCC.

Serum alpha-fetoprotein (AFP) levels are not included in the diagnostic algorithm for HCC as elevated serum AFP may also be seen in patients with chronic liver disease without HCC such as acute or chronic viral hepatitis [9]. However, it is accepted that serum AFP levels greater than 500 µg/L, in a high-risk patient, are diagnostic of HCC [10]. Serum AFP has also emerged as an important prognostic marker in patients being evaluated for liver transplant. An AFP level >1000 µg/L is associated with a high risk for disease recurrence following transplant [11].

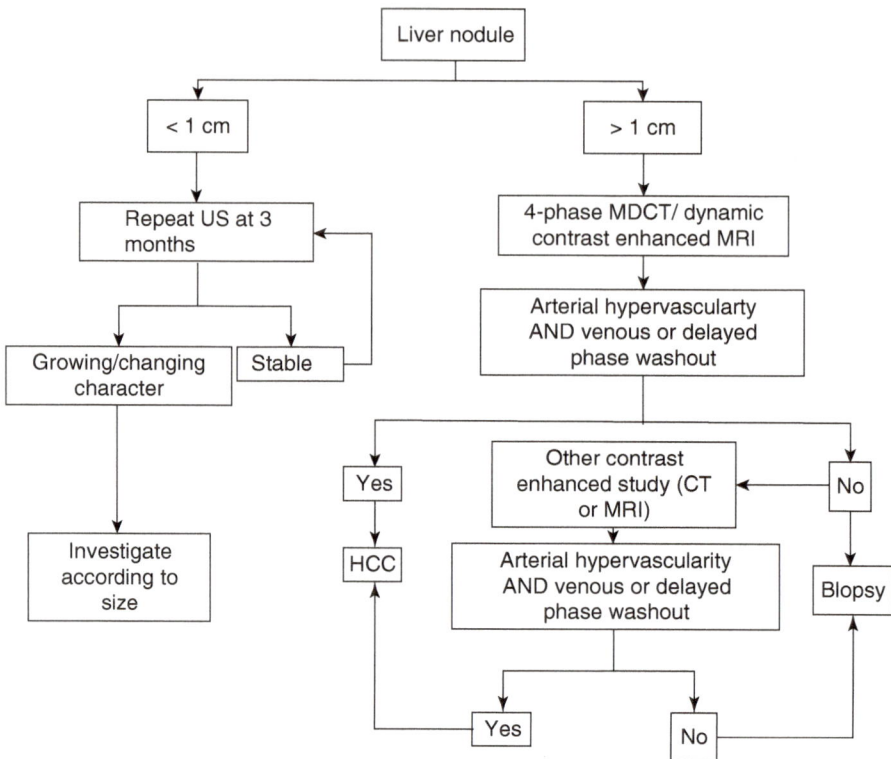

Fig. 1.1 AASLD algorithm for suspected hepatocellular carcinoma [8]. *CT* computed tomography, *MDCT* multidetector CT, *MRI*, magnetic resonance imaging, *US* ultrasonography

The most common sites of extrahepatic metastases in HCC are the lungs, abdominal lymph nodes, and bones, in that order. A CT chest is recommended for all patients being considered for curative resection. On account of low diagnostic yield a bone scan is only recommended for symptomatic patients.

Table 1.3 shows the TNM staging for HCC [12].

1.3 Carcinoma of the Gall Bladder and Bile Ducts

1.3.1 Epidemiology and Etiology

The incidence of gall bladder cancer shows a wide degree of geographical variation with the highest incidence recorded in parts of South America, India, Pakistan, Japan, and Korea [13]. The majority of patients with carcinoma of the gall bladder have gall stone disease. However, the incidence of gall bladder cancer in patients with gall stone disease is just 0.5–3% [14]. Table 1.4 lists the risk factors for gall bladder cancer.

Cholangiocarcinoma arises from the bile duct epithelium and has been classified as intra- and extrahepatic based on anatomical location. Extrahepatic cholangiocarcinomas

Table 1.3 Hepatocellular carcinoma—TNM staging [12]

Primary tumor (T)	
TX	Primary tumor cannot be assessed
T0	No evidence of primary tumor
T1	Solitary tumor without vascular invasion
T2	Solitary tumor with vascular invasion or multiple tumors not more than 5 cm
T3a	Multiple tumors more than 5 cm
T3b	Single tumor or multiple tumors of any size involving a major branch of the portal vein or hepatic vein
T4	Tumor(s) with direct invasion of adjacent organs other than the gallbladder or with perforation of visceral peritoneum
Regional lymph nodes (N)	
NX	Regional lymph nodes cannot be assessed
N0	No regional lymph node metastasis
N1	Regional lymph node metastasis
Distant metastasis (M)	
M0	No distant metastasis
M1	Distant metastasis

Anatomic stage/prognostic groups			
Stage I	T1	N0	M0
Stage II	T2	N0	M0
Stage IIIA	T3a	N0	M0
Stage IIIB	T3b	N0	M0
Stage IIIC	T4	N0	M0
Stage IVA	Any T	N1	M0
Stage IVB	Any T	Any N	M1

Table 1.4 Gall bladder cancer—risk factors

Gallstone disease
Porcelain gallbladder
Gallbladder polyps
Primary sclerosing cholangitis
Chronic infection—salmonella, *Helicobacter*
Congenital biliary cysts—choledochal cysts
Abnormal pancreaticobiliary duct junction
Medications—methyldopa, oral contraceptives, isoniazid
Carcinogen exposure—oil, paper, chemical, shoe, textile industries
Obesity and elevated blood sugar

are further classified as perihilar (up to the insertion of the cystic duct into the bile duct) and distal. Perihilar tumors in turn are further classified as per the Bismuth-Corlette system into four types (Table 1.5) [15]. Hilar cholangiocarcinomas are collectively known as Klatskin tumors.

Table 1.5 Bismuth-Corlette classification of perihilar cholangiocarcinoma [15]

Type 1—Tumors below the confluence of the right and left hepatic ducts

Type 2—Tumors reaching the confluence

Type 3—Tumors involving the confluence and either the right (3a) or left (3b) hepatic ducts

Type 4—Multicentric tumors or those involving the confluence and both the right and left ducts

Primary sclerosing cholangitis and fibropolycystic liver disease (e.g., choledochal cysts) are the major risk factors for cholangiocarcinoma. Intrahepatic cholangiocarcinoma is also associated with chronic liver disease and liver fluke infestation (e.g., clonorchis sinensis). Two familial syndromes, viz., Lynch syndrome and biliary papillomatosis [16], also predispose to cholangiocarcinoma.

1.3.2 Clinical Presentation

Patients with early-stage gall bladder cancer are usually asymptomatic, or present with symptoms of underlying gall stone disease. A large number of early-stage cancers present incidentally on imaging for other indications, or postoperatively, in the histopathology report of cholecystectomy for gall stone disease. Locally advanced disease may present with jaundice due to infiltration of the porta hepatis or compression at the porta due to metastatic lymphadenopathy. Duodenal or colonic obstruction due to a gall bladder primary usually represents inoperable disease.

Extrahepatic cholangiocarcinoma usually presents with biliary tract obstruction as evidenced by jaundice, pruritus, clay-colored stools, and high-colored urine. Associated symptoms include dull aching right hypochondrium pain, malaise, anorexia, and weight loss. Secondary infection of static bile in an obstructed biliary system leads to cholangitis, with a triad of right hypochondrium pain, fever, and jaundice.

Intrahepatic cholangiocarcinomas account for 20% of cases [17] and are largely asymptomatic. Early cases are usually diagnosed incidentally. Large intrahepatic masses may present with vague abdominal pain, anorexia, and weight loss.

1.3.3 Diagnosis and Staging

Ultrasonography is usually the first investigation to evaluate patients with symptoms suggestive of biliary tract pathology. An ultrasound will confirm the presence of biliary tract dilatation, localize the level of block, exclude gall stone disease, and detect metastatic disease in the form of liver metastasis, gross peritoneal deposits, or ascites. Gall bladder polyps more than 1 cm in diameter should be treated with cholecystectomy as they are likely to harbor invasive malignancy [18].

A suspicion of malignancy on ultrasound is further investigated with either a contrast-enhanced CT scan or an MRI. Gall bladder cancer may appear as an intraluminal mass, enhancing wall thickening of the gall bladder, a mass in the gall bladder fossa with or without liver parenchymal infiltration. Biliary ductal dilatation (>6 mm) with enhancing wall thickening is suggestive of cholangiocarcinoma. Intrahepatic cholangiocarcinomas appear as a mass-forming lesion in the liver parenchyma.

Magnetic resonance cholangiopancreatography (MRCP) is particularly useful in patients with biliary tract obstruction, as it will not only accurately delineate the level of obstruction (and type of block) but will also reveal liver metastasis and aberrant bile duct anatomy. Endoscopic retrograde cholangiopancreaticography (ERCP) is useful in distal cholangiocarcinomas with obstructive jaundice, where delineating biliary anatomy and the level of obstruction, obtaining bile/brush cytology and therapeutic stenting, is possible in a single investigation.

Tissue diagnosis is not mandatory for resectable gall bladder masses suspicious for malignancy or for resectable cholangiocarcinomas, but should be obtained if neoadjuvant or palliative treatment is planned. Gall bladder cancers have a predilection for peritoneal seeding, and a percutaneous biopsy/FNAC is preferably avoided in a curative setting. Endoscopic ultrasound (EUS) is a useful tool in gall bladder cancer for characterizing gall bladder polyps, defining depth of wall infiltration, determining lymph node involvement, and obtaining an EUS-guided FNAC.

A baseline Ca 19–9 is obtained for all patients with gall bladder and biliary tract malignancy as it serves as a prognostic indicator with the caveat that biliary obstruction itself may contribute to a raised CA 19–9.

The role of PET scan in gall bladder and biliary tract malignancies is best limited to the detection of occult metastasis [19].

The AJCC TNM system is used for staging gall bladder (Table 1.6) and biliary duct cancers [12]. There are separate staging systems for intrahepatic, perihilar, and distal cholangiocarcinomas.

Table 1.6 TNM staging—gall bladder cancer [12]

Primary tumor (T)	
TX	Primary tumor cannot be assessed
T0	No evidence of primary tumor
Tis	Carcinoma in situ
T1	Tumor invades lamina propria or muscular layer
T1a	Tumor invades lamina propria
T1b	Tumor invades muscular layer
T2	Tumor invades perimuscular connective tissue; no extension beyond serosa or into the liver
T3	Tumor perforates the serosa (visceral peritoneum) and/or directly invades the liver and/or one other adjacent organ or structure, such as the stomach, duodenum, colon, pancreas, omentum, or extrahepatic bile ducts
T4	Tumor invades main portal vein or hepatic artery or invades two or more extrahepatic organs or structures
Regional lymph nodes (N)	
NX	Regional lymph nodes cannot be assessed
N0	No regional lymph node metastasis
N1	Metastases to nodes along the cystic duct, common bile duct, hepatic artery, and/or portal vein
N2	Metastases to periaortic, pericaval, superior mesenteric artery, and/or celiac artery lymph nodes
Distant metastasis (M)	
M0	No distant metastasis
M1	Distant metastasis

1.4   Pancreatic Carcinoma

1.4.1   Epidemiology and Etiology

Worldwide pancreatic cancer is the eighth leading cause of cancer-related deaths in men and the ninth in women [1]. New Zealand Maoris, native Hawaiians, and black Americans have the highest reported incidence [20]. Men are more commonly affected, and the disease is rarely seen before the age of 45 years.

Major risk factors for pancreatic cancer include cigarette smoking, chronic pancreatitis, diabetes mellitus, high body mass index, low physical activity, pancreatic cysts including IPMN (intraductal papillary mucinous neoplasm), and a family history of pancreatic cancer. Pancreatic cancer may also occur in the setting of familial syndromes like hereditary breast and ovarian cancer syndrome, Lynch syndrome, hereditary pancreatitis, Ataxia-telangiectasia, and Li-Fraumeni syndrome.

1.4.2   Clinical Presentation

The clinical presentation of cancer of the exocrine pancreas depends on the location of the tumor within the gland. Sixty to seventy percent of tumors are located in the head, 20–25% in the body and tail, and the rest involves the entire organ [21].

Periampullary and pancreatic head masses usually present with symptoms of obstructive jaundice, viz., yellow discoloration of sclera, clay-colored stools, steatorrhoea, and high-colored urine. Jaundice is usually painless and progressive in nature. A history of waxing and waning jaundice can often be elicited in periampullary tumors.

Pain is a common symptom and is located in the epigastrium with characteristic radiation to the back. Constitutional symptoms of anorexia and weight loss are also common, and recent onset diabetes mellitus could be the first presenting sign [22]. A palpable abdominal mass, free fluid in the abdomen, palpable left supraclavicular node (Virchow's node), and periumbilical nodule (Sister Mary Joseph nodule) are signs of advanced disease.

1.4.3   Diagnosis and Staging

A triple-phase, pancreas protocol, contrast-enhanced, multidetector row CT scan of the abdomen is the gold standard for imaging of pancreatic cancer. A malignant pancreatic mass is typically ill defined and hypodense as compared to the pancreatic parenchyma. Dilatation of the biliary and pancreatic ducts (double duct sign) is present in 62–77% of cases but is not diagnostic of pancreatic head malignancy

[23]. Assessment of resectability with respect to involvement of the superior mesenteric artery (SMA), superior mesenteric vein (SMV), portal vein, coeliac axis, and aorta is made on CT scan.

ERCP is an invasive procedure with a low but defined incidence of mortality (0.2%) and risks of pancreatitis, bleeding, and cholangitis. It is indicated when there is a suspicion of choledocholithiasis and where biliary drainage and stenting are required.

MRCP may be helpful in patients with bulky tumors with duodenal obstruction, in patients with prior gastrectomy (Billroth II) and to detect biliary duct obstruction in the setting of chronic pancreatitis.

Serum levels of CA 19–9 are obtained in all cases of pancreatic cancer as they have prognostic implications [24]. The level of Ca19–9 may also help to predict the possibility of occult metastasis, help in selection of patients for staging laparoscopy, indicate the likelihood of an R0 resection, and give an indication of long-term outcomes [25, 26].

Patients who are fit for major surgery with a resectable mass on CT scan do not require a preoperative biopsy to confirm malignancy. However, in young patients with history of ethanol abuse and in patients with history of other autoimmune diseases, a differential diagnosis of autoimmune pancreatitis should be considered. An EUS in these situations will help to further characterize the pancreatic mass and obtain an EUS-guided FNAC/biopsy. Tissue diagnosis is also mandatory in patients requiring neoadjuvant therapy and in unresectable lesions prior to starting treatment.

The AJCC TNM system is used for staging cancers of the exocrine pancreas [12] (Table 1.7).

Table 1.7 TNM staging—pancreatic cancer [12]

Primary tumor (T)	
TX	Primary tumor cannot be assessed
T0	No evidence of primary tumor
Tis	Carcinoma in situ
T1	Tumor limited to the pancreas, 2 cm or less in greatest dimension
T2	Tumor limited to the pancreas, more than 2 cm in greatest dimension
T3	Tumor extends beyond the pancreas but without involvement of the celiac axis or the superior mesenteric artery
T4	Tumor involves the celiac axis or the superior mesenteric artery (unresectable primary tumor)
Regional lymph nodes (N)	
NX	Regional lymph nodes cannot be assessed
N0	No regional lymph node metastasis
N1	Regional lymph node metastasis
Distant metastasis (M)	
M0	No distant metastasis
M1	Distant metastasis

Key Points

- HCC constitutes the second leading cause of cancer-related deaths in men and the sixth leading cause of cancer-related deaths in women.

- Nearly 80% of HCC cases are due to underlying chronic hepatitis B and C infection.

- Triple-phase contrast-enhanced CT scan or MRI is the investigative modality of choice for HCC.

- The most common sites of extrahepatic metastases in HCC are the lungs, abdominal lymph nodes, and bones.

- The incidence of gall bladder cancer shows a wide degree of geographical variation with the highest incidence recorded in parts of South America, India, Pakistan, Japan, and Korea.

- Primary sclerosing cholangitis and fibropolycystic liver disease are the major risk factors for cholangiocarcinoma.

- Ultrasonography is usually the first investigation to evaluate patients with symptoms suggestive of biliary tract pathology.

- MRCP is useful in patients with biliary tract obstruction.

- Worldwide pancreatic cancer is the eight leading cause of cancer-related deaths in men and the ninth in women.

- A triple-phase, pancreas protocol, contrast-enhanced, multidetector row CT scan of the abdomen is the gold standard for imaging of pancreatic cancer.

References

1. Jemal A, Bray F, Centre MM, et al. Global cancer statistics. CA Cancer J Clin. 2011;61:69.
2. Perz JF, Armstrong GL, Farrington LA, et al. The contributions of hepatitis B virus and hepatitis C virus infections to cirrhosis and primary liver cancer worldwide. J Heptol. 2006;45:529.
3. Beasley RP, Hwang LY, Lin CC, Chien CS. Hepatocellular carcinoma and hepatitis B virus. A prospective study of 22707 men in Taiwan. Lancet. 1981;2:1129.
4. Colombo M, deFranchis R, Del Ninni E, et al. Hepatocellular carcinoma in Italian patients with cirrhosis. N Engl J Med. 1991;325:675.
5. Kew MC, Dos Santos HA, Sherlock S. Diagnosis of primary cancer of the liver. Br Med J. 1971;4:408.
6. Schwartz JM, Larson AM, Gold PJ, et al. Hepatocellular carcinoma: A one year experience at a tertiary referral center in the United States (abstract). Heptatology. 1999;278A:30.
7. A new prognostic system for hepatocellular carcinoma: a retrospective study of 435 patients: the Cancer of the Liver Italian Program (CLIP) investigators. Hepatology 1998;28:751.
8. Bruix J, Sherman M. American Association for the Study of Liver Diseases. Management of hepatocellular carcinoma an update. Hepatology. 2011;53:1020.

9. Sterling RK, Wright EC, Morgan TR, et al. Frequency of elevated hepatocellular carcinoma (HCC) biomarkers in patients with advanced hepatitis C. Am J Gastroenterol. 2012;107:64.
10. Serum WJT. alpha-fetoprotein and its lectin reactivity in liver diseases: a review. Ann Clin Lab Sci. 1990;20:98.
11. Ioannou GN, Perkins JD, Carithers RL Jr. Liver transplantation for hepatocellular carcinoma: impact of the MELD allocation system and predictors of survival. Gastroenterology 2008;134:1342.
12. American Joint Committee on Cancer Staging Manual. 7th, Edge SB, Byrd DR, Compton CC, et al (Eds). New York: Springer; 2010.
13. Randi G, Franceschi S, La Vecchia C. Gall bladder cancer worldwide: geographical distribution and risk factors. Int J Cancer. 2006;118:1591.
14. Carriaga MT, Henson DE. Liver, gallbladder, extrahepatic bile duct, and pancreas. Cancer. 1995;75:171.
15. Bismuth H, Nakache R, Diamond T. Management strategies in resection for hilar cholangiocarcinoma. Ann Surg. 1992;215:31.
16. Lee SS, Kim MH, Lee SK, et al. Clinicopathologic review of 58 patients with biliary papillomatosis. Cancer. 2004;100:783.
17. Saha SK, Zhu AX, Fuchs CS, Brooks GA. Forty-year trends in cholangiocarcinoma incidence in the U.S.: intrahepatic disease on the rise. Oncologist. 2016;21:594.
18. Kubota K, Bandai Y, Noie T, et al. How should polyploidy lesions of the gall bladder be treated in the era of laparoscopic cholecystectomy? Surgery. 1995;117:481.
19. Petrowsky H, Wildbrett P, Husarik DB, et al. Impact of integrated positron emission tomography and computed tomography on staging and management of gall bladder cancer and cholangiocarcinoma. J Hepatol. 2006;45:43.
20. Boyle P, Hseih CC, Maisonneuve P, et al. Epidemiology oc pancreas cancer (1988). Int J Pancreatol. 1989;5:327.
21. Modolell I, Guarner L, Malagelada JR. Vagaries of clinical presentation of pancreatic and biliary tract cancer. Ann Oncol. 1999;10(Suppl 4):82.
22. Aggarwal G, Kamada P, Chari ST. Prevalence of diabetes mellitus in pancreatic cancer compared to common cancers. Pancreas. 2013;42:198.
23. Nino-Murcia M, Jeffrey RB Jr, Beaulieu CF, et al. Multidetector CT of the pancreas and bile duct system: value of curved planar reformations. AJR Am J Roentgenol 2001;176:689.
24. Humphris JL, Chang DK, Johns AL, et al. The prognostic and predictive value of serum Ca 19.9 in pancreatic cancer. Ann Oncol. 2012;23:1713.
25. Karachristos A, Scarmeas N, Hoffman JP. CA 19-9 level predict results of staging laparoscopy in pancreatic cancer. J Gastroinest Surg. 2005;9:1286.
26. Fujioka S, Misawa T, Okamoto T, et al. preoperative serum carcinoembryonic antigen and carbohydrate antigen 19-9 level for the evaluation of curability and resectability in patients with pancreatic adenocarcinoma. J Hepatobiliary Pancreat Surg. 2007;14:539.

Pathology of Hepatobiliary and Pancreatic Cancer

2

Kedar Deodhar

Contents

2.1   Introduction

The prevalence of gastrointestinal (GI) cancers shows a marked geographical variation. These differences can be attributed to many factors including lifestyle, genetics and infection. Globally, colorectum, stomach and liver are the third, fourth and fifth most commonly diagnosed cancers in males, colorectum being the second most common in females [1].

2.2   Gall Bladder

Gall bladder cancer is uncommon in many European countries and the USA and commoner in some countries in Latin America and Asia. The highest incidence occurs in women from Delhi (India) (around 21/100,000) followed by South Karachi, Pakistan and Quito, Ecuador [2].

K. Deodhar
Department of Pathology, Tata Memorial Hospital, Mumbai, Maharashtra, India
e-mail: kedardeodhar@hotmail.com

© Springer International Publishing AG 2018
N. Purandare, S. Shah (eds.), *PET/CT in Hepatobiliary and Pancreatic Malignancies*, Clinicians' Guides to Radionuclide Hybrid Imaging,
DOI 10.1007/978-3-319-60507-4_2

The risk factors for gall bladder cancers have not been clearly identified. However, gall stones are found in more than 80% of the patients with carcinoma and a causal relationship is suggested [3].

Adenoma of the gall bladder is uncommon, but they are the most common benign neoplasms. Adults are affected with a female preponderance. They can measure from 0.5 to 2 cm in diameter and can be sessile or pedunculated. They are usually detected incidentally or while investigating for calculous or acalculous chronic cholecystitis. They are benign lesions and cholecystectomy is curative.

The overall pathogenesis of adenocarcinoma of the gall bladder is thought to result from dysplasia to carcinoma. Metaplasia (gastric, pyloric type and intestinal) are not thought to be premalignant per se. Mutation in the TP53 gene is a common event, and immunohistochemistry (IHC) overexpression of P53 correlates with point mutation.

Grossly, gall bladder carcinomas usually result in localised thickening rather than diffuse thickening. They are mostly located in the body and the fundus (90%) and about 10% are in the neck.

Precursor lesions of adenocarcinomas are termed as biliary intraepithelial neoplasia (low-grade Bil IN 1, 2) and high-grade (Bil IN 3) as in bile ducts [4, 5].

The commonest histological type of cancers of the gall bladder is adenocarcinoma, which accounts for 75–85% of all carcinomas (Fig. 2.1). They can show papillary, tubular architecture and show a variety of cell types such as intestinal,

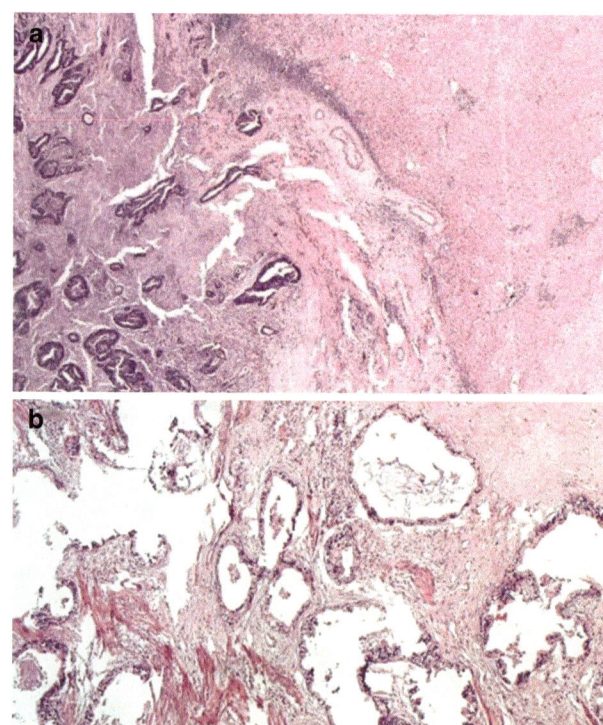

Fig. 2.1 Moderately differentiated adenocarcinoma of the gall bladder. (a) Tumour invades the gall bladder adventitia and is close to liver parenchyma (low power). (b) High-power view of adenocarcinoma

mucinous, clear cell type. Squamous differentiation is commonly seen and can be variable.

Squamous carcinoma, small-cell neuroendocrine carcinoma and undifferentiated carcinoma are some of the uncommon types of carcinomas, each forming upto 3% [4, 6]. Histologically, squamous differentiation in the adenocarcinoma of the gall bladder is common. Hence, diagnosis of a primary squamous carcinoma of the gall bladder is made after extensive sampling and after excluding gland formation as well as any other secondary tumour.

Undifferentiated carcinoma lacks gland formation and can have spindle cells, giant cells and pleomorphic cells. They are very aggressive tumours which frequently metastasize.

The prognosis depends on the stage of the disease.

Nonneoplasic lesion of the gall bladder includes inflammatory polyp, adenomyoma and cholesterol polyps.

Liver cancer is much more common in men than in women. In men, it is the second leading cause of cancer death worldwide and in fewer developing countries [1].

Liver cancer rates are the highest in East and Southeast Asia and Northern and Western Africa. Most primary liver cancers (70–90%) are hepatocellular carcinomas (HCC) (Fig. 2.2). Chronic liver disease and cirrhosis remain the most important risk factors for development of HCC of which viral hepatitis and excessive alcohol intake are the leading risk factors worldwide [7]. Several histological patterns are identified such as clear cell type, adenomatoid, small cell type, etc. Fibro lamellar HCC is a special variant which is seen in young adults and occurs in the liver that are normal. No risk factors are identified for this variant.

Other type of cancers includes cholangiocarcinoma, hepatoblastoma (in younger age) and angiosarcoma.

Cholangiocarcinomas (CC) can have similar histological and immunohistochemical (IHC) profile to that of gall bladder and pancreatic adenocarcinomas. The distinction of cholangiocarcinoma from HCC on a needle-core biopsy can be tricky.

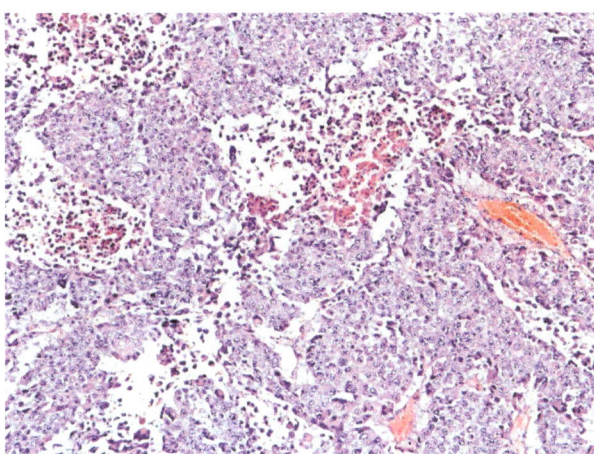

Fig. 2.2 Hepatocellular carcinoma. Histology shows hepatoid tumour cells having rather sheeted appearance and foci of necrosis. No portal triads are seen

HCC are generally immunopositive for Heppar-1 and glypican 3, whereas CC are positive for CK7, CK20 and CK19 and are negative for Heppar-1 and glypican 3. But often, histopathologist looks at clues such as tumour markers (raised alfa feto protein levels versus raised serum Ca19.9/CEA levels) and contrast enhancement in arterial phase on CT scan. Combined hepatocellular and cholangiocarcinoma (CHC) is a recognised entity and accounts for 0.4–14.2% of primary liver cancers. They have overlapping histological features of both HCC and CC [8].

Hepatoblastoma is the most common malignant liver tumour in children and comprises approximately 1% of all paediatric cancers. Nearly 90% of cases occur in the age group of 6 months to 5 years. It is seen typically as a large single mass, occurs in normal livers and almost always shows a marked rise in serum alfa feto protein levels [4]. Histologically, they are of epithelial and mixed epithelial and mesenchymal type and can show cartilage/osteoid, which may give diagnostic clues in imaging. Extramedullary haematopoiesis is often seen in these tumours.

Hepatocellular adenoma is seen mostly in young women during reproductive age and is uncommon in males. They are often solitary and occur in livers that are normal. Long-term use of oral contraceptive pills (OC pills) and use of anabolic steroids are risk factors. Other risk factors include diabetes, glycogen storage diseases types I and IV, tyrosinemia and galactosemia [4]. Hepatic adenoma shows proliferation of hepatocytes with minimal atypia, but with lack of portal zones. The reticulin framework is often maintained. Immunohistochemistry is not helpful in the diagnosis.

Bile duct adenoma is a localised benign ductular proliferation of bile ducts. They are subcapsular in location, smaller than 2 cm in size, and are usually single. They are often sent for frozen section examination to exclude metastatic adenocarcinoma. This can be a difficult diagnosis. Round outline and lack of atypia can point towards this diagnosis.

2.3   Pancreatic Carcinoma

Pancreatic carcinoma is one of the most lethal of all solid malignancies despite therapeutic and research advances. Five-year survival is less than 5% [9].

The incidence rates and mortality rates of pancreatic cancers are generally higher in the USA, Europe, Australia and Japan and lower in India, Africa and parts of Middle East. In India, the age adjusted incidence rate is 1.1/100,000 [10]. More than 95% of pancreatic cancers arise in exocrine portion, whereas about 5% arise in the endocrine portion of the pancreas. The majority are ductal-type adenocarcinomas (Fig. 2.3).

Pancreatic cancer cells, cancer stem cells and tumour microenvironment are the three most crucial components. Pancreatic cancer stem cells (which can comprise of 1–5%) of the total cancer cell population are resistant to chemotherapy. Additionally, the poorly vascularised characteristic pancreatic stroma plays an important role in progression and invasion. Pancreatic stellate cells (also called as myofibroblasts) are a key cellular element in the stroma [11].

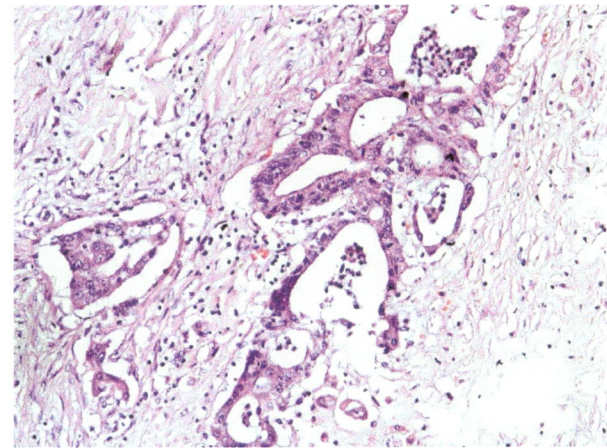

Fig. 2.3 Ductal-type pancreatic adenocarcinoma. Neoplastic glands are irregularly situated in the stroma showing a myxoid and fibrous response

Epidemiological studies looking for aetiology of pancreatic cancers are inconclusive. However, a twofold increase in risk for tobacco smokers is observed than nonsmokers [12].

It is now well established that in the pancreas, similar to colorectal carcinoma, noninvasive precursor lesions of the conventional ductal carcinoma exist. They are termed as pancreatic intraepithelial neoplasia (Pan In). They have been identified from studies of the resected specimens and autopsy studies [13]. The same genes are mutated in Pan Ins as in invasive pancreatic ductal carcinoma.

Pan Ins are microscopic lesions (less than 0.5 cm) and arise in the smaller ducts. They are divided into Pan In1,2 (low grade) and Pan In 3 (high grade). These show increasing degree of nuclear crowding, pseudostratification and hyperchromasia (grade 3 being most severe).

Pan In needs to be distinguished from intraductal pancreatic mucinous neoplasm (IPMN). The latter is the larger mass-forming lesions and can be diagnosed on imaging.

The variants of pancreatic carcinoma include colloid carcinoma (pools of mucin in which atypical mucinous epithelial cells are seen). They almost always arise on the background of intestinal type of IPMN and exhibit intestinal differentiation evident by CDX-2 (transcription factor regulating intestinal programming) and MUC2 (goblet cell type of intestinal mucin). They have a significantly better prognosis than conventional ductal adenocarcinomas [4].

Medullary carcinoma is a distinct subtype of pancreatic carcinoma characterised by poor differentiation, syncytial growth pattern, pushing borders and Crohn's-like lymphoid infiltrate. Most of these tumours are MSI (microsatellite instability) high tumours. IHC can play a role in identifying this subtype, as MSI high tumours have a better prognosis and predict poor response to 5FU-based chemotherapy.

Other pancreatic carcinoma types are undifferentiated carcinoma and acinar carcinoma.

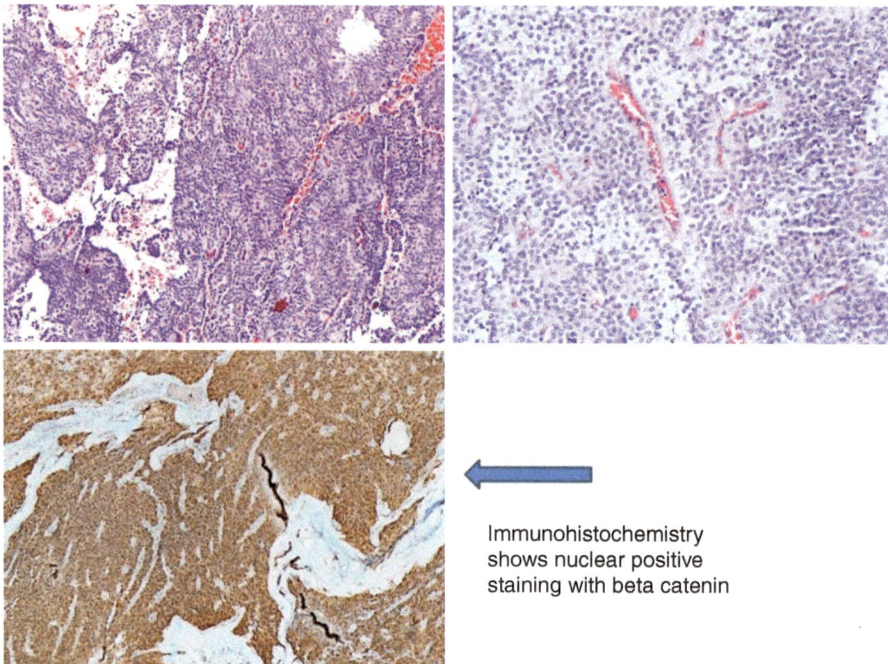

Immunohistochemistry
shows nuclear positive
staining with beta catenin

Fig. 2.4 Solid pseudopapillary tumour of the pancreas (SPEN). Histology shows pseudopapillae lined by relatively uniform cells. Immunohistochemistry shows nuclear beta catenin positivity

Mucinous cystic neoplasm is a cystic tumour lined by mucinous epithelium and ovarian-type stroma. They arise in premenopausal women (female to male ratio 201:1) but can be seen in males as well. They involve pancreatic tail more often than the head. The epithelium shows increasing grades of dysplasia.

Solid pseudopapillary tumour of the pancreas (SPEN) is a distinct neoplasm seen in younger females. It is a slow growing tumour and has a favourable prognosis. Surgery is curative (Fig. 2.4).

Key Points

Gall Bladder

• The overall pathogenesis of adenocarcinoma of the gall bladder is thought to result from dysplasia to carcinoma.

• In general, gall bladder carcinomas usually result from localised thickening rather than diffuse thickening. They are mostly located in the body and the fundus (90%) and about 10% are in the neck.

- The commonest histological type of cancers of the gall bladder is adeno-carcinoma, which accounts for 75–85% of all carcinomas.

- Squamous carcinoma, small-cell neuroendocrine carcinoma and undifferentiated carcinoma are some of the uncommon types.

Liver Cancer

- Most primary liver cancers (70–90%) are hepatocellular carcinomas (HCC). Several histological patterns are identified such as clear cell type, adenomatoid, small cell type, etc.

- Fibro lamellar HCC is a special variant which is seen in young adults and occurs in the liver that is normal.

- Cholangiocarcinomas (CC) can have similar histological and immunohistochemical (IHC) profile to that of gall bladder and pancreatic adenocarcinomas.

- Combined hepatocellular and cholangiocarcinoma (CHC) is a recognised entity and accounts for 0.4–14.2% of primary liver cancers.

Pancreatic Carcinoma

- The majority are ductal-type adenocarcinomas.

- It is now well established that in the pancreas, similar to colorectal carcinoma, noninvasive precursor lesions of the conventional ductal carcinoma exist.

- Medullary carcinoma is a distinct subtype of pancreatic carcinoma.

- Mucinous cystic neoplasm is a cystic tumour lined by mucinous epithelium and ovarian-type stroma.

- Solid pseudopapillary tumour of the pancreas (SPEN) is a distinct neoplasm seen in younger females. It is a slow growing tumour and has a favourable prognosis.

References

1. Torre LA, Bray F, Siegel RL, Farley J, Lortet-Tieulent J, Jemal A. Global cancer statistics, 2012. CA Cancer J Clin. 2015;65:87–108.
2. International Agency for Research on Cancer. World cancer report. Lyon: International Agency for Research on Cancer; 2008.
3. Mathur AV. Need for prophylactic cholecystectomy in silent gall stones in North India. Indian J Surg Oncol. 2014;6:251–5.

4. Farrell L, Kakar S. Tumors of the liver, biliary tree and gall bladder. In: Fletcher CDM , editor. Diagnostic histopathology of tumours, vol. 1. 4th ed. Philadelphia: Elsevier Saunders; 2013.
5. Kloppel G, Adsay V, Konukiewitz B, Kleeff J, Schlitter AM, Esposito I. Precancerous lesions of the biliary tree. Best Pract Res Clin Gastroenterol. 2013;2:285–97.
6. Chandana M, Pant L, Garg M, Singh G, Singh S. Primary pure keratinising squamous carcinoma: a rare malignancy with aggressive behaviour. J Clin Diagn Res. 2016;10:CD21–2.
7. Balogh J, Victor D III, Asham E, Gordon S, Burroughs SG, Boktour M, et al. Hepatocellular carcinoma: a review. J Hepatocellular Carcinoma. 2016;3:41–53.
8. Wang AQ, Zheng YC, Du J, Zhu CP, Huang HC, Wang SS, et al. Combined hepatocellular cholangiocarcinoma: controversies to be addressed. World J Gastroenterol. 2016;22:4459–65.
9. Jemal A, Siegel R, Ward E, Murray T, Xu J, Smigal C et al. Cancer Statistics 2006. CA Cancer J Clin. 2006;56:106–30.
10. National Cancer Registry Programme. Three year report of population based Cancer registries 2006-2008: Incidence of distribution of Cancer. Bengaluru: Indian Council of Medical Research; 2010.
11. Rucki AA, Zheng L. Pancreatic cancer stroma: understanding biology leads to new therapeutic strategies. World J Gastroenterol. 2104;20:2237–46.
12. Iodice S, Gandini S, Maisonneuve P, Lowenfels AB. Tobacco and the risk of pancreatic cancer: a review and meta-analysis. Langenbecks Arch Surg. 2008;393:535–45.
13. Basturk O, Hong SM, Wood LD, Adsay NV, Albores-Saavedra J, Biankin AV, et al. A revised classification system and recommendations from the Baltimore Consensus Meeting for Neoplastic Precursor Lesions in the Pancreas. Am J Surg Pathol. 2015;39:1730–41.

Management of Hepatobiliary and Pancreatic Malignancies

3

Ashwin deSouza

Contents

3.1 Introduction

Surgery plays an integral role and perhaps offers the only curative option in the management of hepatobiliary and pancreatic malignancies. Chemotherapy and radiation, either in the neoadjuvant or adjuvant setting, have further complemented the outcomes of radical surgery and play an important role in palliation. This chapter presents the principles of management of hepatocellular carcinoma (HCC), cancers of the gall bladder and biliary tract and pancreatic cancer.

A. deSouza, M.S., M.Ch., M.R.C.S.Ed., D.N.B
Department of Gastrointestinal and HPB Surgery, Tata Memorial Centre,
Mumbai, Maharashtra, India
e-mail: ashwindesouza@gmail.com

© Springer International Publishing AG 2018
N. Purandare, S. Shah (eds.), *PET/CT in Hepatobiliary and Pancreatic Malignancies*, Clinicians' Guides to Radionuclide Hybrid Imaging, DOI 10.1007/978-3-319-60507-4_3

3.2   Management of HCC

Surgical resection forms the mainstay in the treatment of HCC. However, the majority of patients are inoperable at presentation either on account of tumour extent or underlying liver dysfunction.

Estimation of liver functional status by the Child-Turcotte-Pugh classification forms the backbone of estimation of liver functional reserve (Table 3.1).

There are various treatment options in the management of HCC as listed below. Decisions on treatment strategy are best taken on an individual basis through a multidisciplinary approach.

1. Surgical resection
2. Liver transplantation
3. Radiofrequency ablation (RFA)
4. Transarterial chemoembolization (TACE)
5. Radioembolization
6. Radiotherapy and stereotactic radiotherapy
7. Systemic chemotherapy and targeted therapy

1. Surgical Resection
   Patients ideally suited for surgical resection are those who have disease limited to the liver, with no radiographic evidence of invasion of the liver vasculature, well-preserved liver function (Child's A) and no portal hypertension [1–3]. Preoperative evaluation is best done with a multidisciplinary team to document adequate volume and function of the residual liver remnant. CT volumetry gives an accurate estimation of residual liver volume, and indocyanine green clearance is often used to estimate liver functional status in patients with borderline liver function. Long-term overall survival rates of $\geq 40\%$ can be achieved with limited hepatic resections for small tumours (<5 cm) in patients with Child-Pugh class A cirrhosis [4].

Table 3.1 Liver functional status—Child-Turcotte-Pugh classification

	Points assigned		
Parameter	1	2	3
Ascites	Absent	Slight	Moderate
Bilirubin	<2 mg/dL	2–3 mg/dL	>3 mg/dL
Albumin	>3.5 g/dL	2.8–3.5 g/dL	<2.8 g/dL
Prothrombin time (seconds over control) (INR)	<4 (<1.7)	4–6 (1.7–2.3)	>6 (>2.3)
Encephalopathy	None	Grade 1–2	Grade 3–4

A total Child-Turcotte-Pugh score of 5–6 is considered Child-Pugh class A (well-compensated disease); 7–9 is class B (significant functional compromise); and 10–15 is class C (decompensated disease). *INR* international normalized ratio

2. Liver Transplantation

   For patients with localized HCC who are not candidates for resection, orthotopic liver transplantation is indicated in single lesions ≤5 cm, up to three separate lesions, not larger than 3 cm, no evidence of gross vascular invasion and no regional nodal or extrahepatic distant metastases. When these criteria are applied, a 4-year survival rate of 75% can be achieved. These criteria have become known as the Milan criteria and have been widely applied around the world in the selection of patients with HCC for liver transplantation [5].

3. Radiofrequency Ablation

   This technique uses high-frequency radio waves to ablate the tumour and is best suited for deep-seated small lesions (<3 cm) situated away from the hepatic hilum. The approach can be offered for tumours up to 5 cm and is associated with a local recurrence rate of 5–20%. Local ablation with RFA is recommended for patients who cannot undergo surgery or as a bridge to transplantation.

4. TACE

   Transarterial chemoembolization is indicated in patients with unresectable HCC that is multifocal or too large for percutaneous ablation, relatively preserved liver function (Child-Pugh A or B) and no extrahepatic disease, vascular invasion or portal vein thrombosis. TACE has been shown to provide a survival advantage over supportive care only in randomized trials [6, 7]. It is also used as a bridge to liver transplant.

5. Radioembolization

   Transarterial radioembolization (TARE) involves the transarterial administration of microspheres labelled with yttrium-90 (Y-90), which is a beta ray emitter having a half-life of 64.2 h and a maximum tumour penetration of 10 mm. These microspheres have a diameter of <60 μm and therefore have the ability to be shunted to the lungs or abdominal viscera. Elaborate pretreatment planning is required which includes mesenteric angiography, dosimetry planning and a transarterial macro-aggregated albumin study to look for pulmonary shunting. Transarterial radioembolization is usually preferred in the setting of portal vein thrombosis as it is associated with less embolic events [8]. Data from retrospective studies also show a trend towards better downstaging prior to transplant.

6. Radiotherapy and Stereotactic Radiotherapy

   Although HCC is a radiosensitive tumour, it is located in an extremely radiosensitive organ. Three-dimensional conformal radiation (3D–CRT) and stereotactic body radiotherapy techniques deliver higher doses of radiation to the tumour with less liver toxicity as compared to conventional radiotherapy. There is a lack of consensus as to appropriate indications for RT in patients with HCC. However, 3D–CRT or SBRT is a reasonable option for selected patients who are being considered for other local treatment modalities and have no extrahepatic disease, limited tumour burden and relatively preserved liver function (Child-Pugh class A or early class B).

7. Systemic Chemotherapy and Targeted Therapy

Hepatocellular carcinoma is a relatively chemotherapy-refractory tumour. Although data suggests some antitumour activity of a number of chemotherapeutic agents, their use is preferable within the context of a clinical trial. Sorafenib is an oral multikinase inhibitor that has shown activity in HCC. In 2007, it was approved for treatment of unresectable HCC by the United States FDA. This was based on data from randomized trials [9, 10] which showed a modest improvement in overall survival with sorafenib. Presently, sorafenib can be recommended in unresectable HCC in Child's A and in a select group of Child's B patients.

3.3   Management of Cancers of the Gall Bladder and Bile Duct

3.3.1   Surgery: Gall Bladder Cancer

Surgical resection offers the only potentially curative therapy for gall bladder cancer [11]. Surgery is indicated in Stage 0–II, i.e. Tis, T1, T2, N0 where it may be curative. Periaortic, pericaval, superior mesenteric artery and/or coeliac lymph node involvement (i.e. N2 disease) has a prognosis similar to patients with distant metastasis. This group constitutes unresectable disease (Table 3.2).

For T1a tumours, i.e. invading the lamina propria without muscular layer involvement, a simple cholecystectomy is adequate and offers cure rates of 73–100% [12, 13]. Patients diagnosed with incidental T1a gall bladder carcinoma after a laparoscopic cholecystectomy do not require re-resection as it does not offer any survival advantage [14].

Lymph node metastasis occurs in 15 and 62% of patients with T1b and T2 tumours, respectively [15, 16]. These patients benefit from extended or radical cholecystectomy which involves resection of the gall bladder with an en masse liver wedge resection and periportal lymphadenectomy. An intraoperative frozen section of the cystic duct margin is mandatory. Failure to achieve a negative margin at the cystic duct or frank involvement of the extrahepatic bile duct warrants an extrahepatic biliary tract excision with hepaticojejunostomy. An incidental diagnosis of T1b/T2 gall bladder cancer after simple cholecystectomy warrants a re-resection or revision radical cholecystectomy.

Stage III and Stage IVa, i.e. tumours involving adjacent organs like the stomach, duodenum colon, pancreas and the extrahepatic biliary tree, may be resectable in a

Table 3.2 Gall bladder cancer—criteria for inoperability

Liver metastasis
Peritoneal metastasis
Involvement of N2 nodes (coeliac, peripancreatic, periduodenal, superior mesenteric nodes)
Malignant ascites
Extensive involvement of the hepatoduodenal ligament (infiltration of branches of the hepatic artery or portal vein)
Presence of distant metastasis

selected group of patients. Surgery in this situation entails en masse resection of the involved organs and is best reserved for the fit patient at a high volume centre. Although prognosis remains guarded for this group of patients, retrospective series report favourable survival for these patients if an R0 resection can be achieved [17, 18]. However, the majority of Stage IVa tumours have involvement of the hepatic artery or portal vein rendering them unresectable. There is no role for debulking surgery; surgical exploration should only be undertaken if an R0 resection is feasible.

3.3.2   Surgery: Cholangiocarcinoma

Although surgery offers the only option for long-term control of cholangiocarcinoma, the 5-year survival rates are very poor, especially for node-positive disease even if an R0 resection is achieved. Resectability rates depend not only on tumour location but equally on the available surgical expertise as these are very specialized surgical procedures. Resectability rates for distal, intrahepatic and perihilar lesions have been reported as 91%, 60% and 56%, respectively [19].

Intrahepatic cholangiocarcinomas are managed by a formal hepatic resection and distal cholangiocarcinomas are resected with a pancreaticoduodenectomy. Perihilar tumours are the most surgically challenging. Even at high volume centres, resectability rates are less than 50%. Resection of the extrahepatic bile ducts alone leads to high rates of local recurrence either at the confluence of the hepatic ducts or at the caudate lobe branches. Addition of a hepatectomy with a caudate lobectomy improves outcomes [20, 21]. The type of surgical resection depends on the Bismuth subtype. For type I and II tumours, the procedure involves an en bloc resection of the extrahepatic ducts (with a 5–10 mm margin) with the gall bladder, regional lymphadenectomy and hepaticojejunostomy. A hepatic lobectomy is often required to achieve adequate margins on the bile ducts. Type III lesions usually require an additional lobectomy or trisectionectomy. As the caudate lobe branches are frequently involved in type II and III tumours, most centres recommend a caudate lobectomy in these patients. Extended resections involving the portal vein and/or multiple hepatic resections can be offered for the select few with type III and IV tumours at centres of excellence [22].

3.3.3   Adjuvant Therapy: Gall Bladder Cancer

T3 and/or node-positive gall bladder cancer is associated with poor survival outcomes even if an R0 resection is achieved. This suggests a role for adjuvant chemotherapy/radiation therapy. High quality data for adjuvant chemotherapy in gall bladder cancer is scarce, and hence participation in clinical trials is recommended.

Adjuvant chemotherapy is recommended for tumours ≥T2, node-positive disease and/or margin-positive resection. Generally, 6 months of adjuvant chemotherapy is recommended using gemcitabine, 5-fluorouracil (5-FU) or a combination of both. Alternatively, 5-FU based chemoradiotherapy along with systemic chemotherapy is another acceptable option [23]. This regimen may be particularly beneficial for patient with margin-positive resection where systemic chemotherapy followed by chemoradiotherapy is recommended.

3.3.4   Adjuvant Therapy: Cholangiocarcinoma

The evidence to support the routine administration of adjuvant therapy in resected cholangiocarcinoma is scarce, leading to a variety of available options in different patient groups.

Intrahepatic cholangiocarcinoma with a margin negative resection and no residual disease can be observed. Adjuvant chemotherapy, chemoradiotherapy, re-resection (if feasible) and ablation are acceptable options for margin-positive intrahepatic cholangiocarcinoma. Extrahepatic cholangiocarcinoma resected with negative margins and negative nodes may be observed. Alternatively some centres recommend adjuvant chemoradiotherapy or systemic chemotherapy for these patients. Margin-positive resections may benefit from adjuvant chemoradiation followed by systemic chemotherapy, and node-positive disease warrants adjuvant systemic chemotherapy. Wherever applicable, systemic chemotherapy for cholangiocarcinoma is either fluoropyrimidine or gemcitabine based.

3.3.5   Unresectable Disease: Gall Bladder Cancer and Cholangiocarcinoma

The management of locally advanced and unresectable carcinoma of the gall bladder and bile ducts is essentially palliative barring a few exceptions. The goals of management of these patients are relieving of obstructive jaundice, pain relief and prolongation of life. Jaundice is effectively palliated with self-expanding metallic stents placed within the occluded bile ducts either via percutaneous, transhepatic or endoscopic route. In patients of good performance status, systemic chemotherapy, chemoradiotherapy or a combination of both are acceptable options. These patients are at high risk to develop metastatic disease; therefore, a treatment regimen beginning with systemic chemotherapy followed by chemoradiotherapy for the patients with good response and absence of metastatic disease is probably the most appropriate. Palliative chemotherapy (gemcitabine/cisplatin/fluoropyrimidine based) remains the only option for fit patients with metastatic disease.

3.4   Management of Pancreatic Cancer

Only 15–20% of patients with pancreatic cancer are resectable at initial presentation. Key to the surgical management of pancreatic cancer is the initial classification of pancreatic tumours into resectable, borderline resettable and unresectable disease. The National

Table 3.3 Borderline resectable and unresectable pancreatic cancer—National Comprehensive Cancer Network (NCCN) definitions

Tumour location	Criteria
Unresectable pancreatic cancer	
Pancreatic head/ uncinate lesions	Tumour contact with SMA / Coeliac axis > 180 degrees
	Solid tumour contact with the first jejunal branch of the SMA / SMV
	Non-reconstructable SMV/portal vein involvement
Pancreatic body and tail lesions	Tumour contact with SMA / Coeliac axis greater than 180°
	Non-reconstructable SMV/portal vein involvement
	Aortic involvement
For all sites	Distant metastasis
	Lymph node metastasis beyond the surgical field of dissection
Boderline Resectable pancreatic cancer	
For tumours of the head or uncinate process	Solid tumour contact with SMV/portal vein >180 degrees, allowing for safe and complete resection and vein reconstruction
	Less than one-half the circumference (180°) of tumour abutment on the SMA
	Abutment or encasement of the hepatic artery, if reconstructable. Solid tumour contact with variable anatomy e.g accessory right hepatic artery.
	Solid tumour contact with the IVC
For tumours of the body and tail	Less than 180° contact of the tumour with the SMA or coeliac axis

Comprehensive Cancer Network (NCCN) has defined borderline resectable and unresectable pancreatic cancer for tumours at different locations in the gland (Table 3.3).

The choice of surgical procedure depends on tumour location. Tumours in the pancreatic head and periampullary region are resected with a pancreaticoduodenectomy. A pylorus-preserving procedure is preferred wherever feasible as it leads to better functional outcomes without compromise on oncological adequacy [24]. A pylorus-preserving pancreaticoduodenectomy will remove the entire duodenum (sparing the first 3–4 cm distal to the pylorus), the pancreatic head, uncinate process, proximal jejunum and peripancreatic and hepatoduodenal lymph nodes. Reconstruction is achieved with either a pancreaticogastrostomy or pancreaticojejunostomy, a hepaticojejunostomy and a duodenojejunostomy.

Patients presenting with obstructive jaundice and with either bilirubin above 20 mg/dL or with signs of cholangitis or in those in whom surgery will be delayed for more than 2 weeks undergo preoperative biliary drainage either endoscopically with endoscopic retrograde cholangio-pancreaticography (ERCP) and biliary stenting or via the percutaneous transhepatic approach. Preoperative biliary drainage while associated with a higher incidence of postoperative complications [25] may be beneficial in this select group of patients.

Tumours in the body and tail of the pancreas are best managed with a subtotal or distal pancreatectomy with or without a splenectomy. Rarely a total pancreatectomy is necessary to surgically extirpate disease diffusely involving the entire gland.

Neoadjuvant therapy is the first line of management for borderline resectable tumours. Neoadjuvant chemotherapy (gemcitabine/fluoropyrimidine based), fluoropyrimidine-based chemoradiotherapy or both are acceptable options. A large proportion of borderline resectable tumours undergo R0 resection following neoadjuvant therapy with encouraging outcomes [26, 27].

Unresectable but non-metastatic pancreatic cancer is treated with initial chemotherapy (gemcitabine/nabpaclitaxel/FOLFIRINOX (5-FU + leucovorin + irinotecan + oxaliplatin)) followed either by fluoropyrimidine-based chemoradiation or further chemotherapy to maximal response.

Adjuvant chemotherapy is recommended for all patients following pancreatic resection [28, 29]. Gemcitabine with or without capecitabine for a duration of 6 months after recovery from surgery is the recommended protocol. Patients with node-positive disease and/or margin-positive resections may receive additional chemoradiotherapy following adjuvant chemotherapy [29].

Key Points

- Decisions on treatment strategy are best taken on an individual basis through a multidisciplinary approach.

- Surgery plays an integral role and perhaps offers the only curative option in the management of hepatobiliary and pancreatic malignancies.

- Surgical resection forms the mainstay in the treatment of HCC. However, the majority of patients are inoperable at presentation.

- *Radiofrequency ablation in HCC is* best suited for deep-seated small lesions (<3 cm) situated away from the hepatic hilum. Local ablation with RFA is recommended for patients who cannot undergo surgery or as a bridge to transplantation.

- *TACE is* indicated in patients with unresectable HCC that is multifocal or too large for percutaneous ablation, relatively preserved liver function (Child-Pugh A or B) and no extrahepatic disease, vascular invasion or portal vein thrombosis.

- Adjuvant chemotherapy is recommended for gall bladder tumours ≥T2, node-positive disease and/or margin-positive resection.

- The management of locally advanced and unresectable carcinoma of the gall bladder and bile ducts is essentially palliative barring a few exceptions.

- Only 15–20% of patients with pancreatic cancer are resectable at initial presentation. The choice of surgical procedure depends on tumour location. Pylorus preserving pancreaticoduodenectomy is the procedure of choice for resectable tumours in the pancreatic head and uncinate process.

- Tumours in the body and tail of the pancreas are best managed with a subtotal or distal pancreatectomy with or without a splenectomy.

- Adjuvant chemotherapy is recommended for all patients following pancreatic resection.

References

1. Bruix J. Treatment of hepatocellular carcinoma. Hepatology. 1997;25:259.
2. Vauthey JN, Klimstra D, Franceschi D, et al. Factors affecting long-term outcome after hepatic resection for hepatocellular carcinoma. Am J Surg. 1995;169:28.
3. Bruix J, Castells A, Bosch J, et al. Surgical resection of hepatocellular carcinoma in cirrhotic patients: prognostic value of preoperative portal pressure. Gastroenterology. 1996;111:1018.
4. Roayaie S, Obeidat K, Sposito C, et al. Resection of hepatocellular cancer ≤2cm: results from two western centers. Hepatology. 2013;57:1426.
5. Mazzaferro V, Regalia E, Doci R, et al. Liver transplantation for the treatment of small hepatocellular carcinomas in patient with cirrhosis. N Engl J Med. 1996;334:693.
6. Lo CN, Ngan H, Tsa WK, et al. Randomized controlled trial of transarterial lipiodol chemoembolization for unresectable hepatocellular carcinoma. Hepatology. 2002;35:1164.
7. Llovet JM, Real MI, Montana X, et al. Arterial embolisation or chemoembolisation versus symptomatic treatment in patients with unresectable hepatocellular carcinoma: a randomized controlled trial. Lancet. 2002;359:1734.
8. Salem R, Lewandowski RJ, Mulcahy MF, et al. Radioembolisation for hepatocellular carcinoma using yttrium-90 microspheres: a comprehensive report of long-term outcomes. Gastroenterology. 2010;138:52.
9. Llovet JM, Ricci S, Mazzaferro V, et al. Sorafenib in advanced hepatocellular carcinoma. N Engl J Med. 2008;359:378–90.
10. Cheng AL, Kang YK, Chen Z, et al. Efficacy and safety of sorafenib in patients in the Asia-Pacific region with advanced hepatocellular carcinoma: a phase III randomised, double-blind, placebo-controlled trial. Lancet Oncol. 2009;10:25–34.
11. Jayaraman S, Jarnagin WR. Management of gall bladder cancer. Gastroenterol Clin North Am. 2010;39:331.
12. Shirai Y, Yoshida K, Tsukada K, et al. Early carcinoma of the gall bladder. Eur J Surg. 1992;158:545.
13. Wakai T, Shirai Y, Yokoyama N, et al. Early gall bladder carcinoma does not warrant radical resection. Br J Surg. 2001;88:675.
14. You DD, Lee HG, Paik Ky, et al. What is an adequate extent of resection for T1 gall bladder cancers? Ann Surg 2008;247:835.
15. Matsumoto Y, Fujii H, Aoyama H, et al. Surgical treatment of primary carcinoma of the gall bladder based on the histologic analysis of 48 surgical specimens. Am J Surg. 1992;163:239.
16. Shimada H, Endo I, Togo S, et al. The role of lymph node dissection in the treatment of gall bladder carcinoma. Cancer. 1997;79:892.
17. Nimura Y, Hayakawa N, Kamiya J, et al. Hepatopancreatoduodenectomy for advanced carcinoma of the biliary tract. Hepatogastroenterology. 1991;38:170.
18. Nakamura S, Suzuki S, Konno H, et al. Outcome of extensive surgery for TNM stage IV carcinoma of the gall bladder. Hepatogastroenterology. 1999;46:2138.
19. Nakeeb A, Pitt HA, Sohn TA, et al. Cholangiocarcinoma. A spectrum of intrahepatic, perihilar and distal tumours. Ann Surg. 1996;224:463.
20. Lim JH, Choi GH, Choi SH, et al. Liver resection for Bismuth type I and type II hilar cholangiocarcinoma. World J Surg. 2013;37:829.
21. Tan JW, Hu BS, Chu YJ et al. one-stage resection for Bismuth type IV hilar cholangiocarcinoma with high hilar resection and parenchyma-preserving strategies: a cohort study. World J Surg 2013;37:614.
22. Hemming AW, Mekeel K, Khanna A, et al. Portal vein resection in management of hilar cholangiocarcinoma. J Am Coll Surg. 2011;212:604.
23. Ben-Josef E, Guthrie KA, El-Khoueiry AB, et al. SWOG S0890: a phase II intergroup trial of adjuvant capecitabine and gemcitabine followed by radiotherapy and concurrent capecitabine in extrahepatic cholangiocarcinoma and gall bladder carcinoma. J Clin Oncol. 2015;33:2617.
24. Diener MK, Knaebel HP, Heukaufer C, et al. A systematic review and meta-analysis of pylorus-preserving versus classical pancreaticoduodenectomy for surgical treatment of periampullary and pancreatic carcinoma. Ann Surg. 2007;245:187.

25. Van de Gaag NA, Rauws EA, van Eijck CH, et al. Preoperative biliary drainage for cancer of the head of pancreas. N Engl J Med. 2010;362:129.
26. Barugola G, Partelli S, Crippa S, et al. Outcomes after resection of locally advanced or borderline resectable pancreatic cancer after neoadjuvant therapy. Am J Surg. 2012;203:132.
27. McClaine RJ, lowry AM, Sussman JJ, et al. Neoadjuvant therapy may lead to successful surgical resection and improved survival in patients with borderline resectable pancreatic cancer. HPB (Oxford) 2010;12:73.
28. Seufferlein T, Bachet JB, Van Cutsem E, et al. Pancreatic adenocarcinoma: ESMO-ESDO clinical practice guidelines for diagnosis, treatment and follow-up. Ann Oncol. 2012;23(Suppl 7):vii33.
29. Khorana AA, Mangu PB, Berlin J, et al. Potentially curable pancreatic cancer: American society of clinical oncology clinical practice guidelines. J Clin Oncol. 2016;34:2541.

Radiological Imaging in Hepatobiliary and Pancreatic Malignancies

4

Suyash Kulkarni, Kunal Gala, Nitin Shetty, and Ashwin Polnaya

Contents

Liver malignancies are briefly divided into hypo- and hypervascular lesions. The lesions in hypovascular groups include metastasis from colon, lung, gastric, prostate and transitional cell carcinomas [1, 2] and cholangiocarcinoma. The hypervascular lesions include hepatocellular carcinoma (HCC) and hypervascular metastasis from breast, melanoma, renal, thyroid and neuroendocrine tumour [2, 3].

HCC is the fifth most common malignant neoplasm worldwide and most common liver malignancy. The risk factors for HCC include hepatitis B, C viral infection, alcoholic cirrhosis, cirrhosis from steatohepatitis and hemochromatosis. Clinical presentation would be non-specific; however, it may have right upper quadrant pain, hepatomegaly, ascites and weight loss. Alpha-fetoprotein (AFP) would be elevated with patients with HCC, and it is used for initial diagnosis and monitoring response to treatment [4], but one third of patients will not have elevation of AFP [5].

With the advancement in imaging, it can provide definite diagnosis; however in atypical or equivocal cases, biopsy needs to be done [6–8].

S. Kulkarni (✉) • K. Gala • N. Shetty • A. Polnaya
Department of Radiology, Tata Memorial Centre, Mumbai, Maharashtra, India
e-mail: suyashkulkarni@yahoo.com

© Springer International Publishing AG 2018
N. Purandare, S. Shah (eds.), *PET/CT in Hepatobiliary and Pancreatic Malignancies*, Clinicians' Guides to Radionuclide Hybrid Imaging,
DOI 10.1007/978-3-319-60507-4_4

HCC

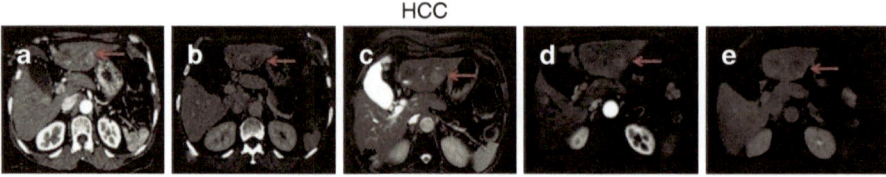

Fig. 4.1 HCC: (**a, b**) contrast-enhanced CT reveals arterially enhancing lesion in the lateral segment, i.e. segment III (**a**), and wash out on porto-venous phases (**b**). On MRI (**c–e**), a well-defined T2 hyperintense signal lesion (**c**) which shows rapid wash in on the arterial phase (**d**) and wash out on porto-venous phase (**e**). These imaging findings are classical for hepatocellular carcinoma

Ultrasound (USG) is the first modality when patient experiences right upper quadrant pain. USG would demonstrate coarse nodular liver with irregular nodular surface, with small shrunken right lobe, hypertrophy of the lateral segments and caudate lobe of the liver, ascites, splenomegaly and varices. HCC would be capsulated hypoechoic lesion when <5 cm [9]. Colour Doppler will demonstrate high-velocity signals and portal vein thrombosis [10] (Fig. 4.1).

The typical pattern of enhancement on both CT and MRI scan would be rapid arterial enhancement and wash-out on porto-venous phases and delayed enhancing capsule due to fibrous nature [11]. Arterio-portal shunting is also one of the characteristic features [12]. HCC can cause spontaneous haemorrhage, and surface HCC can rupture leading to hemoperitoneum. On MR imaging it will be hypointense on T1-weighted imaging. It can be hyperintense due to fat, protein or blood content within. On T2 these lesions would be hyperintense with restricted diffusion. Small HCC are <2 cm in size and have classical features, whereas large HCC will not show classical enhancement pattern and will have haemorrhage and necrosis. HCC are known to cause portal vein tumour thrombus which on imaging will enlarge the portal vein, cause arterial enhancement and neovascularity. HCC can have scar, calcification, fat and blood and can be cystic. They can be solitary, well-defined, multiple or diffuse [13].

Fibrolamellar carcinoma occurs in younger patients without underlying liver disease. These on imaging appear as large well-defined lobulated tumours with central scar, calcifications and heterogeneous enhancement [14, 15]. On MRI, these are hypointense on T1-weighted and heterogeneously hyperintense on T2-weighted images [15]. The scar is hypointense on T2 and shows delayed enhancement on post-contrast.

LI-RADS—The Liver Imaging Reporting and Data System is developed by the American College of Radiology with the aim to reduce variability in lesion interpretation, standardizing of the reporting content, improving communication with the clinician and decision-making, outcome monitoring, performance auditing, quality assurance and research [16].

Biopsy is indicated for the nodules which are >1 cm and do not show characteristic pattern on imaging [17–19].

BCLC staging is widely used for HCC since it combines predictor of survival and treatment options.

BCLC staging is widely used for HCC since it combines predictor of survival and treatment options. In radiological stage B of BCLC which is an intermediate group, say, one lesion more than 3 cm or more than three lesions irrespective of size, the best option is transarterial chemoembolization (TACE) [20].

Other liver lesions are discussed in the table.

Liver tumours	Imaging findings
Metastases	On imaging these will be solitary or multiple and well defined which may be hypervascular as in renal cell carcinoma, carcinoid tumour, malignant adrenal tumours, thyroid carcinoma, pancreatic islet cell tumours, NET, sarcomas and melanomas. Calcifications can occur in mucinous colon carcinoma and gastric, breast, renal, carcinoid and lung carcinomas. On MR, these will be hypointense on T1 and hyperintense on T2, except for haemorrhagic lesions which have T1-hyperintense lesions (Fig. 4.2)
Biliary cystadenocarcinoma	On CT these are well-defined intrahepatic masses, which are cystic, with enhancing wall, mural, septal nodules or soft tissue papillary projections on contrast study. On MRI, T1 and T2 show variable signal intensity but will have contrast enhancement similar to CECT
Haemangioendothelioma	Middle age, predominant in females. Lesions are multiple which coalesce to form masses, capsular retraction; tumour enhances peripherally. On MR, hypointense on T1 and homogenous or heterogeneously hyperintense on T2 with peripheral enhancement
Angiosarcoma	Variable enhancement which may be nodular and irregular; may have areas of haemorrhage within. On MR, large mass which may be hypo or hyper due to haemorrhage on T1 and heterogeneously hyperintense on T2 and may show heterogeneous and progressive enhancement on post-contrast

For MRI contrast agents for the liver. There are four types:

1. Extracellular agents
2. Reticuloendothelial agents
3. Hepatobiliary agents
4. Blood pool agents
5. Combined agents

Metastasis

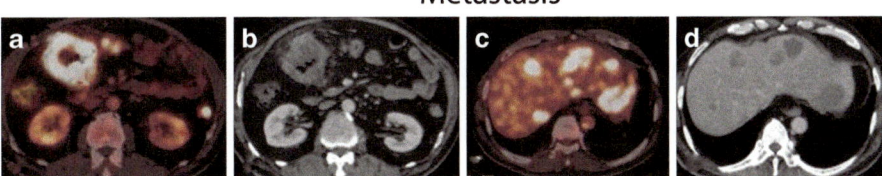

Fig. 4.2 Metastasis: Sixty-year old gentleman with pain in abdomen and mild constipation for 3 months. USG reveals multiple hypoechoic lesions. The above PET/CT images reveals FDG avid lesion in the hepatic flexure (**a**) which on corresponding CECT reveals circumferential heterogeneously enhancing thickening (**b**). Also FDG avid hepatic lesions (**c**) which on CECT (**d**) shows non-enhancing liver lesions. Colonoscopy and biopsy were done which reveal adenocarcinoma

Extracellular agents—Mechanism depends on the gadolinium, which has seven unpaired electrons and is highly paramagnetic resulting in shortening of the T1 and T2 relaxation times of adjacent water protons and causing signal enhancement at T1-weighted imaging and loss of signal at T2-weighted imaging [21, 22]. It is used in lesion detection, characterization and liver vascular anatomy.

Reticuloendothelial agents—Superparamagnetic iron oxides, e.g. ferucarbotran, are currently used as reticuloendothelial agents. They are phagocytosed by macrophages throughout the body but are entrapped by Kupffer cells [23]. They act as negative contrast agent, and due to their superparamagnetic properties, they cause T2 and T2 * shortening [24]. It is used with liver tumours since they are deficient in Kupffer cells and do not exhibit SPIO particle uptake. So after injection of SPIO, the tumour will appear hyperintense since the background is suppressed [25].

Hepatobiliary agents—As they have five unpaired electrons, paramagnetic agents are taken by functioning hepatocytes and excreted in the bile [26]. It shortens T1 and T2 relaxation times of water protons. It is used for characterization of hepatocellular and non-hepatocellular masses since these agents are taken by the hepatocytes (e.g. HCC, focal nodular hyperplasia, hepatic adenoma) and surveillance of the liver for metastasis and functioning of biliary system.

Combined agents—Gadobenate dimeglumine has the property of an extracellular, hepatobiliary and blood pool agent. It is used for HCC, focal nodular hyperplasia and non-hepatocellular lesions, adenoma, metastasis and haemangioma [26].

Cholangiocarcinoma is the second most common malignancy of the biliary system. According to its anatomical origin, it is classified as intrahepatic, hilar or extrahepatic [27].

Intrahepatic CC is an adenocarcinoma that arises from the epithelium of the small intrahepatic bile ducts. Predisposing factors are primary sclerosing cholangitis, *Clonorchis sinensis* infestation, thorium dioxide exposure and congenital biliary anomalies. They are further macroscopically divided into mass form, periductal or intraductal growth. Clinical presentation depends on the location of the mass; peripheral masses are diagnosed late as they cause pain only in late stage where central hilar will cause painless jaundice early. On CT it presents as having a low attenuation mass with incomplete peripheral arterial enhancement that becomes iso- or hypodense on porto-venous phase. Capsular retraction is seen due to fibrosis. There can be ductal dilatation and mural thickening seen in peripheral intrahepatic ducts [28]. On MRI they appear hypointense on T1 and hyperintense on T2. Central area may be hypo or hyper due to fibrosis, mucin or oedema. It shows mild to moderate enhancement with progressive centripetal fill-in of the contrast on delayed phases [29]. On USG it shows solid heterogeneous echotexture mass (Fig. 4.3).

Peripheral CC are primary biliary tumours arising between the right and left and the common hepatic duct up to the cystic duct insertion and also known as Klatskin's tumours [30]. On CT/MR, it will show focal mural thickening with luminal obliteration and peripheral ductal dilatation, periductal thickening with mass, focal liver atrophy, vascular encasement, lymph nodal involvement and distant metastasis.

Cholangiocarcinoma

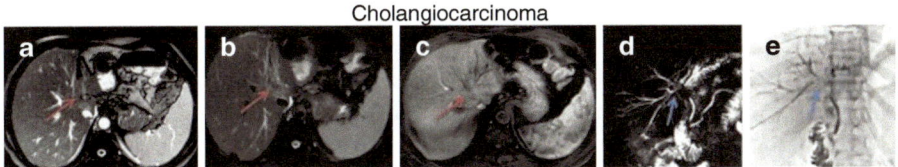

Fig. 4.3 Cholangiocarcinoma: Fifty-eight-year old male with pain in abdomen and progressive painless jaundice since 2 months. CECT done outside reveals mass in the left hepatic duct with periportal lymph nodes. MRI abdomen (**a–c**) with MRCP (**d**) done which shows ill-defined altered signal intensity mass lesion in the left hepatic duct (↗) extending into the common hepatic duct which shows delayed progressive enhancement, atrophy of the left lobe of liver and mild IHBR dilatation in both lobes. These features are s/o cholangiocarcinoma. MRCP (**d**) reveals stricture (↑) involving the left hepatic duct, confluence and just extending into the right anterior and posterior ductal system s/o type IV block. PTC gram (**e**) done which reveals multiple segmental block s/o type IV block

Distal CC originates between the insertion of the cystic duct in the extrahepatic channel and the ampulla of Vater. On cross-sectional imaging, tumour will show soft tissue density with delayed enhancement and abrupt cut-off and infiltrative thickening of bile duct wall.

4.1 Gall Bladder Carcinoma

It is the most common biliary malignancy worldwide. Most of the patients are diagnosed in late stages due to vague symptoms. Predisposing factors include cholelithiasis, porcelain gall bladder, choledochal cyst, congenital cystic dilatation of biliary tree, anomalous pancreatico-biliary junction and low cystic duct insertion and primary sclerosing cholangitis. Clinical presentation includes abdominal pain, fever, weight loss and jaundice [31].

There are three patterns of gall bladder carcinoma:

1. Mass obliterating the gall bladder lumen
2. Focal or diffuse gall bladder wall thickening
3. Intraluminal polypoidal mass [32]

Radiological features in:

1. Mass-forming lesion—On USG it shows heterogeneously hypoechoic mass filling partially or completely. On CT it will show heterogeneously enhancing mass lesion. There may be presence of calcification within the mass or calculi within the gall bladder lumen [33]. On MRI it will show T1 hypointensity and T2 moderate hyperintensity. Similar contrast enhancement is seen as that of CT. CT helps to demonstrate involvement of the hepatic flexure of the colon or regional adenopathy. Primary tumour can infiltrate along the bile ducts and biliary system.
2. Focal or diffuse wall thickening—On cross-sectional imaging, it will show asymmetrical, irregular or extensive thickening showing heterogeneous

enhancement. It needs to be differentiated from acute and chronic cholecystitis, xanthogranulomatous cholecystitis and adenomyomatosis.

3. Intraluminal polypoidal mass—It is a mass larger than 1 cm in diameter which is immobile upon changing position on USG.

CT scan is for preoperative staging and MRCP for bile duct and vascular invasion.

4.2   Pancreatic Carcinoma

Pancreatic adenocarcinoma is the most common malignancy of the pancreas.

These tumours are located 60–70% in the pancreatic head, 10–20% in the pancreatic body and 5–10% in the pancreatic tail. They present with pain in abdomen, weight loss and jaundice.

On ultrasound it would be a poorly defined heterogeneous hypoechoic mass. Other indirect signs include dilatation of the pancreatic duct, biliary duct dilatation or both (double duct sign). On CT it will be hypoenhancing mass; tumour in the pancreatic head causes dilatation of CBD and main pancreatic duct, whereas tumour in body of pancreas will cause upstream MPD dilatation. Cross-section imaging will also demonstrate vascular invasion, thrombosis and collateral vessels [34]. On MR it is hypointense on T1 and T2 due to scirrhous fibrotic nature and shows restricted diffusion. Metastases are frequently seen in liver and peritoneum (Fig. 4.4).

Ca pancreas

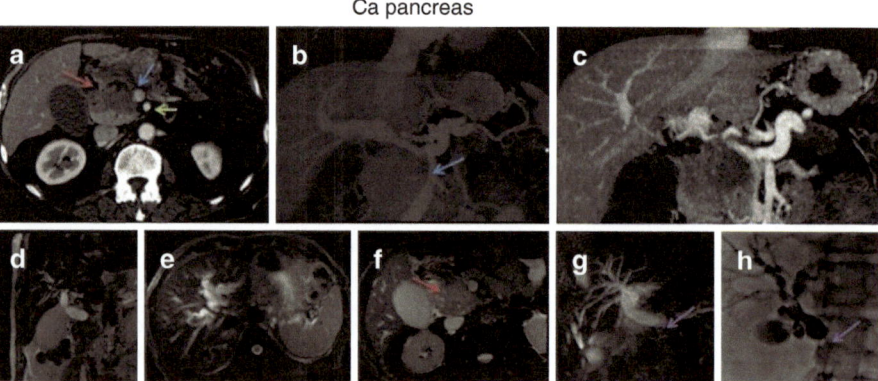

Fig. 4.4 Pancreatic cancer: Seventy-year old male with painless jaundice, weight loss. CECT (**a**, **b**, **c**) reveals mass in the head of pancreas (*red arrow*) with abutting SMV (*blue arrow*) = 180° and SMA (*green arrow*) free with double duct sign and multiple periportal lymph nodes. This is s/o head of pancreas malignancy. MRI abdomen (**d–f**) with MRCP. (**g**) Mass in the head of pancreas (*red arrow*) which shows hyperintense signal on T2 W and shows heterogeneous post contrast enhancement. MRCP shows stricture (*purple arrow*) involving distal common bile duct s/o type I block. PTC gram (**h**) reveals similar findings

One of the newer modality is endoscopic USG, which has similar findings of USG.

FDG-PET shows high metabolic activity in pancreatic adenocarcinoma. Sensitivity and specificity of FDG-PET (96% and 78%, respectively) were superior to those of CT (91% and 56%), transabdominal US (91% and 50%) and endoscopic US (96% and 67%) [35].

NCCN Guidelines for the Resectability of Pancreatic Adenocarcinoma
Resectable

- -No distant metastasis
- -No SMV/PV abutment, distortion, tumour thrombus, venous encasement
- -Clear fat planes around celiac, SMA, HA

Borderline Resectable

- No distant metastasis
- Venous involvement of SMV or PV consisting of tumour abutting with or without impingement and narrowing of the vessel lumen
- Short-segment venous occlusion resulting from either tumour thrombus or encasement but with suitable vessel proximal and distal to the area of tumour involvement, allowing safe resection and reconstruction
- Gastroduodenal artery encasement up to the HA with either short-segment encasement or direct abutment of the HA, without extension to the CA
- Tumour abutment of the SMA $\leq 180°$ of the circumference of the vessel wall

Unresectable
Pancreatic Head
• Distant metastases
• SMA encasement >180°, any CA abutment
• Unreconstructible occlusion of the SMV or PV
• Aortic invasion or encasement
Pancreatic Body
• Distant metastases
• SMA/CA encasement of >180°
• Unreconstructible occlusion of SMV or PV
• Aortic invasion or encasement
Pancreatic Tail
• Distant metastases
• SMA/CA encasement >180°
Nodal status
• Metastases to lymph nodes beyond field of resection [36]

Pancreatic neuroendocrine tumour is solid and shows homogenous enhancement, whereas larger tumour shows heterogeneous, cystic-necrotic degeneration and calcification [37]. On MRI these show hypointense signal on T1 and iso- to hyperintense signal on T2. Metastases to the lymph nodes and liver have similar enhancement as primary tumour.

Other tumours include solid pseudopapillary tumour, cystic pancreatic neoplasm, pancreatic lymphoma and metastasis.

Pancreatic tumour	Imaging findings
Serous cystadenoma	Age—seventh decade. Female more than male, asymptomatic. On CT, multicystic, more than six septated by fibrous septae, lobulated, water, soft tissue density, cysts <2 cm, and hallmark feature is central stellate scar which may contain calcification [38]. On MR cluster of tiny cysts with high signal on T2 with intervening septa and scar
Mucinous cystic neoplasms	Age—fifth and sixth decade. Female more than male; body and tail location. Uniloculated or multiloculated cystic mass > 5 cm. On CT, few and large cysts. Walls may be irregular, contains nodularity or septations and may contain peripheral calcification in 15% [39]
Intraductal papillary mucinous neoplasm	Age—seventh decade. Arises from three types of ductal system—main duct, side branch and mixed. On CT, diffuse or segmental dilatation of the main pancreatic duct. On MR, diffuse or segmental dilatation which will be hypointense on T1 and hyperintense on T2. If there are mural nodules, focal solid area, enhancement of the duct wall and main pancreatic duct diameter of 18 mm [40] may suggest features of malignant transformation of main duct IPMN. Similarly, side-branch IPMN. Features that may suggest malignant transformation: mural nodule, solid component, <3 cm
Pancreatic neuroendocrine tumour	Functioning (secretory) and non-functioning (non-secretory). Small tumours, solid and homogenous, and large tumours, heterogeneous cystic-necrotic and calcification. On MR these have low signal on T1 and intermediate to high signal on T2. These enhance avidly [37]

Key Points

- Liver malignancies are briefly divided into hypo and hypervascular lesions.

- Classical HCC on cross-sectional imaging would show rapid arterial enhancement and wash out on portovenous phases and delayedly enhancing capsule due to fibrous nature, in addition on MRI T2 hyperintensity and restricted diffusion.

- LIRADS- Liver Imaging- Reporting and Data System- aim to reduced variability in the lesion interpretation, standardizing of the reporting content, improving communication with the clinician and decision making, outcome monitoring, performance auditing, quality assurance and research.

- Intra hepatic CC- low attenuation mass with capsular retraction, ductal dilatation and mural thickening seen in peripheral intrahepatic ducts and shows mild to moderate enhancement with progressive centripetal fill-in of the contrast on delayed phases.

- Gall cancer has 3 patterns mass obliterating the gall bladder lumen, focal or diffuse gall bladder wall thickening and intraluminal polypoidal mass.

- Pancreatic cancer on cross section imaging hypoenhancing mass, tumour in pancreatic head with dilatation of CBD and main pancreatic duct (double duct sign).

References

1. Nino-Murcia M, Olcott EW, Jeffrey RB Jr, et al. Focal liver lesions: pattern-based classification scheme for enhancement at arterial phase CT. Radiology. 2000;215:746–51.
2. Danet IM, Semelka RC, Leonardou P, et al. Spectrum of MRI appearances of untreated metastases of the liver. AJR Am J Roentgenol. 2003;181:809–17.
3. Quillin SP, Atilla S, Brown JJ, et al. Characterization of focal hepatic masses by dynamic contrast enhanced MR imaging: findings in 311 lesions. Magn Reson Imaging. 1997;15:275–85.
4. Johnson PJ. The role of serum alpha-fetoprotein estimation in the diagnosis and management of hepatocellular carcinoma. Clin Liver Dis. 2001;5:145–59.
5. Schwarz RE, Smith DD. Trends in local therapy for hepatocellular carcinoma and survival outcomes in the US population. Am J Surg. 2008;195:829–36.
6. Bruix J. Sherman M; Practice Guidelines Committee American Association for the Study of Liver Diseases. Management of hepatocellular carcinoma. Hepatology. 2005;42:1208–36.
7. Mitchell DG, Bruix J, Sherman M, Sirlin CB. LI-RADS (Liver Imaging Reporting and Data System): summary, discussion, and consensus of the LI-RADS Management Working Group and Future Directions. Hepatology. 2015;61:1056–65.
8. Bruix J, Sherman M, Llovet JM, et al. European Association for the Study of the liver. Clinical management of hepatocellular carcinoma: conclusions of the Barcelona-2000 EASL conference. J Hepatol. 2001;35:421–30.
9. Tanaka S, Kitamura T, Imaoka S, et al. Hepatocellular carcinoma: Sonographic and histologic correlation. AJR Am J Roentgenol. 1983;140:701–7.
10. Tanaka S, Kitamura T, Fujita M, et al. Colour Doppler flow imaging of liver tumours. AJR Am J Roentgenol. 1990;154:509–14.
11. Lee JH, Lee JM, Kim SJ, et al. Enhancement patterns of hepatocellular carcinomas on multiphasic multidetector row CT: comparison with pathological differentiation. Br J Radiol. 2012;85:e573–83.
12. Okuda K, Musha H, Yamasaki T, et al. Angiographic demonstration of hepatocellular intra hepatic arterio-portal anastomoses in hepatocellular carcinoma. Radiology. 1977;122:53–8.
13. Becker-Weidman DJ, Kalb B, Sharma P, et al. Hepatocellular carcinoma lesion characterization: single-institution clinical performance review of multiphase gadolinium-enhanced MR imaging-comparison to prior same-center results after MR systems improvements. Radiology. 2011;261: 824–33.
14. DJ B, Johnson CD, Stephens DH, et al. Imaging of fibrolamellar hepatocellular carcinoma. AJR Am J Roentgenol. 1988;151:295–9.
15. McLarney JK, Rucker PT, Bender GN, et al. Fibrolamellar carcinoma of the liver: radiologic-pathologic correlation. Radiographics. 1999;19:453–71.
16. Purysko AS, Remer EM, Coppa CP, Leão Filho HM, Thupili CR, Veniero JC. LI-RADS: A case-based review of the new categorization of liver findings in patients with end-stage liver disease. Radiographics. 2012;32:1977–95. American College of Radiology. Quality and safety resources: Liver Imaging–Reporting and Data System. Available at: https://www.acr.org/Quality-Safety/Resources/LIRADS. Accessed April 22, 2012
17. Bruix J, Sherman M. American Association for the Study of Liver Diseases. Management of hepatocellular carcinoma: an update. Hepatology. 2011;53(3):1020–2.

18. European Association For The Study Of The Liver, European Organisation for Research and Treatment of Cancer. EASL-EORTC clinical practice guidelines: management of hepatocellular carcinoma. J Hepatol. 2012;56(4):908–43.
19. Omata M, Lesmana LA, Tateishi R, et al. Asian Pacific Association for the Study of the Liver consensus recommendations on hepatocellular carcinoma. Hepatol Int. 2010;4(2):439–74.
20. Llovet JM, Bruix J. Systematic review of randomized trials for unresectable hepatocellular carcinoma: chemoembolization improves survival. Hepatology. 2003;37(2):429–42.
21. Semelka RC, Helmberger TK. Contrast agents for MR imaging of the liver. Radiology. 2001;218:27–38.
22. Mitchell DG. Liver I Currently available gadolinium chelates. Magn Reson Imaging Clin N Am. 1996;4:37–51.
23. Schuhmann-Giampieri G. Liver contrast media for magnetic resonance imaging: interrelations between pharmacokinetics and imaging. Investig Radiol. 1993;28:753–61.
24. Ferrucci JT, Stark DD. Iron oxide-enhanced MR imaging of the liver and spleen: review of the first 5 years. AJR Am J Roentgenol. 1990;155:943–50.
25. Kim YK, Kwak HS, Kim CS, Chung GH, Han YM, Lee JM. Hepatocellular carcinoma in patients with chronic liver disease: comparison of SPIO-enhanced MR imaging and 16-detector row CT. Radiology. 2006;238:531–41.
26. Reimer P, Schneider G, Schima W. Hepatobiliary contrast agents for contrast-enhanced MRI of the liver: properties, clinical development and applications. Eur Radiol. 2004;14:559–78.
27. Han JK, Choi BI, Kim AY, An SK, Lee JW, Kim TK, et al. Cholangiocarcinoma: pictorial essay of CT and cholangiographic findings. Radiographics. 2002;22:173–87.
28. Valls C, Guma A, Puig I, et al. Intrahepatic peripheral cholangiocarcinoma: CT evaluation. Abdom Imaging. 2000;25:490–6.
29. Fan ZM, Yamashita Y, Harada M, et al. Intrahepatic cholangiocarcinoma, spin-echo and contrast enhanced dynamic MR imaging. AJR Am J Roentgenol. 1993;161:313–7.
30. Blechacz B, Komuta M, Roskams T, Gores GJ. Clinical diagnosis and staging of cholangiocarcinoma. Nat Rev Gastroenterol Hepatol. 2011;8:512–22.
31. Reid KM, Ramos-De la Medina A, Donohue JH. Diagnosis and surgical management of gallbladder cancer: a review. J Gastrointest Surg. 2007;11:671–81.
32. Levy AD, Murakata LA, Rohrmann CA. Gallbladder carcinoma: radiologic–pathologic correlation. Radiographics. 2001;21:295–314.
33. Franquet T, Montes M, Ruiz de Azua Y, Jimenez FJ, Cozcolluela R. Primary gallbladder carcinoma: imaging findings in 50 patients with pathologic correlation. Gastrointest Radiol. 1991;16:143–8.
34. Ros PR, Mortele KJ. Imaging features of pancreatic neoplasms. JBR-BTR. 2001;84(6):239–49.
35. Inokuma T, Okamoto T, Ogami T, et al. Diagnosis of pancreatic cancer with FDG-PET: comparison with CT, US and endoscopic US. Gut. 1996;39(suppl 3):12.
36. Tempero M, Arnoletti JP, Behrman S, et al. Clinical Practice Guidelines in Oncology: pancreatic adenocarcinoma. National Comprehensive Cancer. Network. 2010; version 2. Available at https://www.nccn.org/. Accessed July 2010.
37. Noone TC, Hosey J, Firat Z, Semelka RC. Imaging and localization of islet-cell tumours of the pancreas on CT and MRI. Best Pract Res Clin Endocrinol Metab. 2005;19(2):195–211.
38. Sarr MG, Kendrick ML, Nagorney DM, Thompson GB, Farley DR, Farnell MB. Cystic neoplasms of the pancreas: benign to malignant epithelial neoplasms. Surg Clin North Am. 2001;81(3):497–509.
39. Sarr MG, Carpenter HA, Prabhakar LP, et al. Clinical and pathologic correlation of 84 mucinous cystic neoplasms of the pancreas: can one reliably differentiate benign from malignant (or premalignant) neoplasms? Ann Surg. 2000;231(2):205–12.
40. Manfredi R, Graziani R, Motton M, et al. Main pancreatic duct intraductal papillary mucinous neoplasms: accuracy of MR imaging in differentiation between benign and malignant tumors compared with histopathologic analysis. Radiology. 2009;253(1):106–15.

FDG PET/CT: Normal Variants, Artefacts and Pitfalls in Hepatobiliary and Pancreatic Malignancies

5

Nilendu Purandare, Sneha Shah, Archi Agrawal, Ameya Puranik, and Venkatesh Rangarajan

Contents

5.1   Introduction

FDG PET/CT is being increasingly used in the evaluation of biliary tract and pancreatic malignancies. Gall bladder cancer and cholangiocarcinoma constitute biliary tract malignancies. Pancreatic adenocarcinoma is frequently staged using FDG PET/CT. The varying histologies and presentations of these tumours give rise to a wide range of normal appearances on FDG PET/CT. Several treatment options like biliary drainage, stenting, surgery, radiation and chemotherapy are used to treat hepatobiliary and pancreatic cancers which produce various tissue changes and can lead to pitfalls and artefacts on PET/CT. Correct and timely recognition of these tissue changes and associated treatment-related complications is important in avoiding diagnostic pitfalls.

N. Purandare (✉) • S. Shah • A. Agrawal • A. Puranik • V. Rangarajan
Department of Nuclear Medicine and Molecular Imaging, Tata Memorial Centre,
Mumbai, Maharashtra, India
e-mail: nilpurandare@gmail.com

© Springer International Publishing AG 2018   41
N. Purandare, S. Shah (eds.), *PET/CT in Hepatobiliary and Pancreatic Malignancies*, Clinicians' Guides to Radionuclide Hybrid Imaging,
DOI 10.1007/978-3-319-60507-4_5

5.2   Variations in Imaging Appearance Due to Anatomy and Histology

Cholangiocarcinoma can show variable FDG uptake depending upon the anatomic location, growth pattern and histological subtype [1–3]. Lesions that are extrahepatic, infiltrative and mucinous in nature tend to show poor or no FDG concentration and can be difficult to localise on PET studies leading to false-negative results (Fig. 5.1). Dilatation of the biliary tree and its pattern on CT are often indirect signs that reveal the site of the lesion (Fig. 5.2). Images acquired at a delayed time point can also help by augmenting the FDG uptake in the lesion (Fig. 5.2).

Cystic neoplasms of the pancreas include serous cystadenoma, mucinous cystadenoma and intraductal pancreatic neoplasms (IPMN). IMPNs are mucin-producing neoplasms that can be benign or invasive carcinomas, and FDG PET very often is used to differentiate between them [4]. Mucinous nature of these tumours causes poor avidity of FDG on PET studies (Fig. 5.3) more so in patients with a tiny malignant focus.

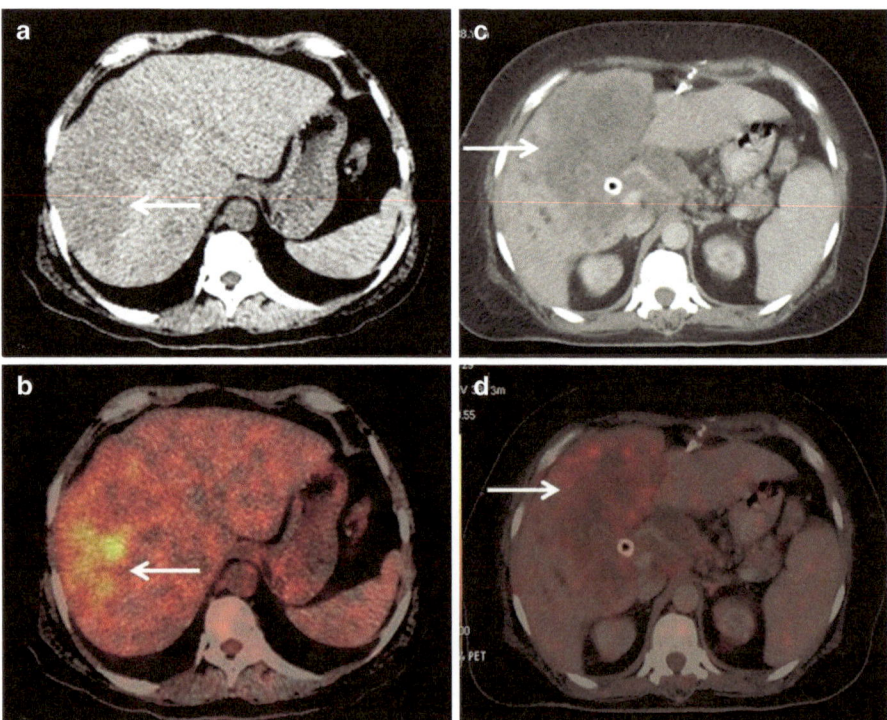

Fig. 5.1 Poor FDG concentrating cholangiocarcinomas. Axial CT and fused PET/CT images shows a diffusely infiltrative type of cholangiocarcinoma showing low-grade FDG uptake (*arrows* in **a**, **b**). Axial CT and fused PET/CT images show extremely poor concentration of FDG in a diffuse mucinous type of cholangiocarcinoma (*arrows* in **c**, d)

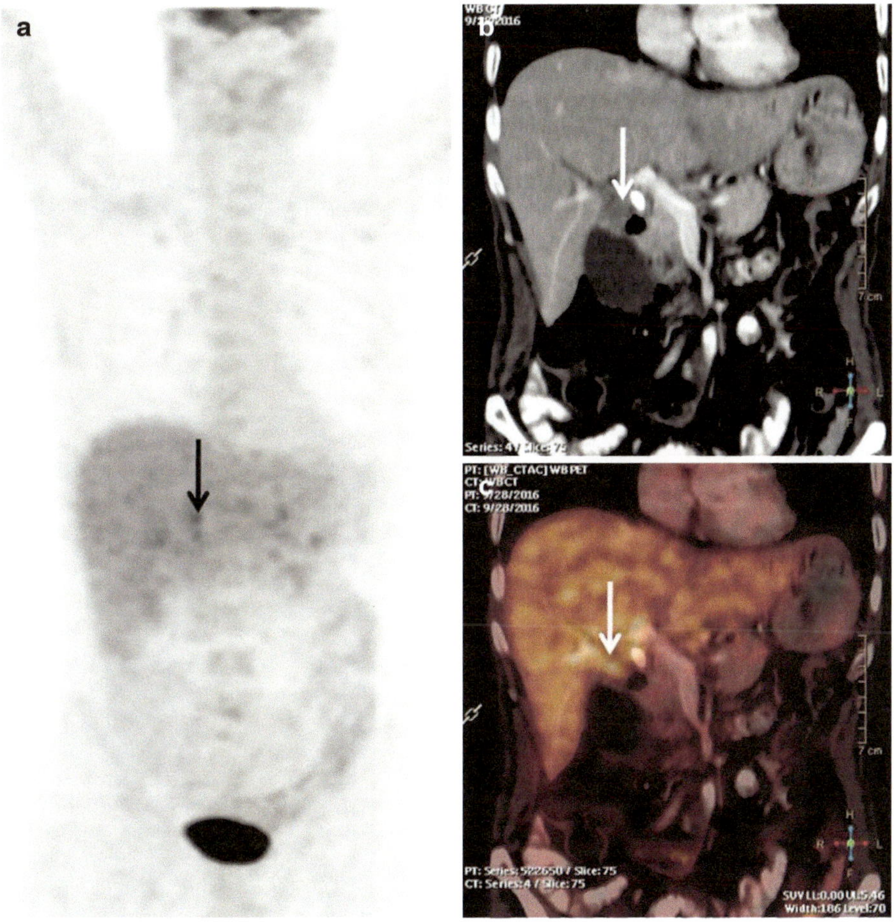

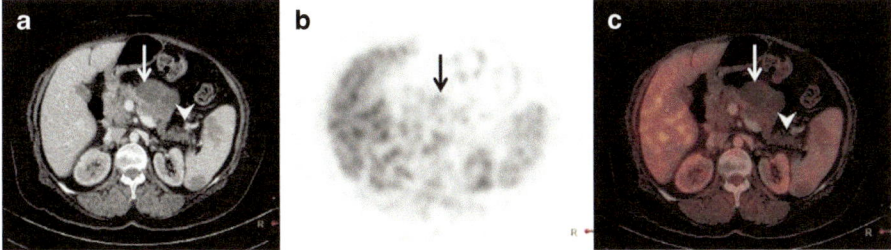

Fig. 5.2 Poor FDG concentrating GB neck and cystic duct malignancy. Coronal MIP and fused PET/CT images (*arrows* in **a, c**) do not show significant FDG concentration in a stricturous lesion involving the neck of the GB and the cystic duct (*arrow* in **b**). Surgical resection revealed a mucin-producing adenocarcinoma

Fig. 5.3 Poor FDG concentration in intraductal papillary mucinous neoplasm of pancreas. Axial CT scan shows a lobulated cystic mass arising from the pancreatic body (*arrow* in **a**) causing atrophy of the distal pancreatic body and tail (*arrowhead* in **a, c**). Axial PET and fused FDG PET/CT reveal no FDG uptake in the lesion. Histopathology after surgical resection showed IPMN with invasive features

5.3   Inflammatory Pathology Mimicking Malignancy

Mass-forming pancreatitis (MFP) resembles pancreatic adenocarcinoma on CT scan, and differentiating one from the other can be challenging. FDG PET/CT has been found to be better in distinguishing MFP from pancreatic adenocarcinoma by virtue of lower tracer uptake in the inflammatory lesion [5, 6]. However, certain cases of MFP can show high FDG avidity due to the inflammatory process and can simulate malignancy (Fig. 5.4).

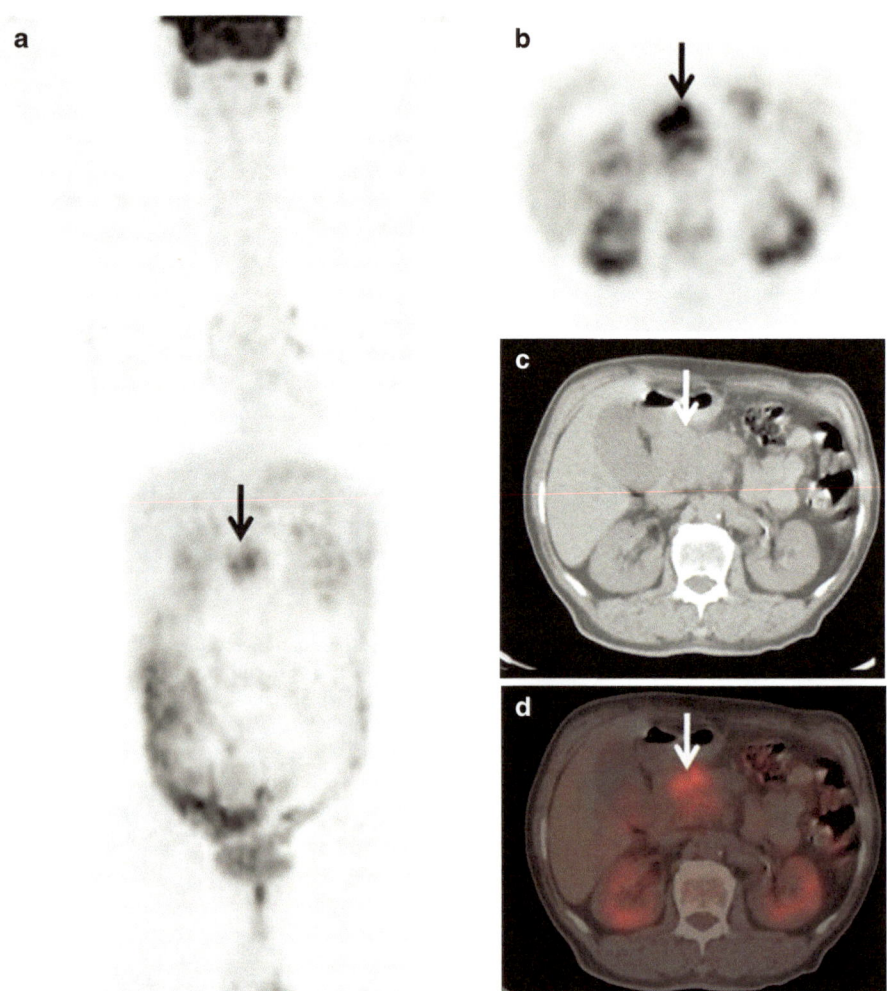

Fig. 5.4 FDG avid mass forming pancreatitis. Coronal MIP, axial PET and fused PET/CT show increased FDG uptake (*arrows* in **a, b, d**) in a soft tissue mass seen in the pancreatic head (*arrow* in **c**). Biopsy revealed pancreatitis. FDG PET can be false positive in mass forming pancreatitis

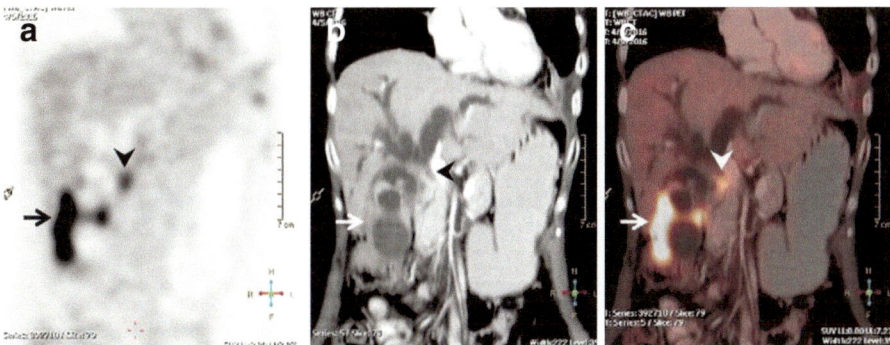

Fig. 5.5 FDG avid cholecystitis. Coronal PET and fusion PET/CT images (*arrowheads* in **a**, **c**) in a biopsy-proven case of cholangiocarcinoma show a FDG avid soft tissue lesion obstructing the common bile duct. FDG uptake along the thickened wall of the gall bladder (*arrows* in **a–c**) is due to cholecystitis and can be erroneously diagnosed as second malignancy

Gall bladder wall thickening can be because of benign causes like inflammation and adenomyosis or due to malignancy. FDG PET can be falsely positive in cases of cholecystitis, and differentiation from malignancy can be difficult [7, 8]. Mass-like or protuberant lesions are more likely to be due to malignancy. Diffuse and uniform FDG avid wall thickening is usually due to inflammation (Fig. 5.5), though imaging features can overlap.

5.4   Pitfalls Due to Treatment-Related Changes and Complications

Significant proportion of gall bladder cancers are diagnosed incidentally from the surgical specimen after elective cholecystectomy is performed for symptomatic calculus disease. Staging PET/CT studies then performed often show FDG uptake in the operated bed of the gall bladder fossa which is due to post-operative inflammation associated with normal healing [2, 9]. This false-positive FDG uptake can persist for several weeks after surgery and mimic disease leading to futile surgical explorations to remove residual disease (Fig. 5.6).

Patients after laparoscopic cholecystectomy for unsuspected gall bladder cancer occasionally develop metastasis at the site of laparoscopy ports. PET/CT can detect port site metastases by demonstrating increased FDG uptake in those regions [10]. Persistent inflammation at the port site causes FDG avidity that can mimic a metastatic deposit (Fig. 5.7). Careful attention should be given to the morphological changes accompanying the metabolic findings. Absence of a nodular soft tissue or a mass lesion at the port site favours an inflammatory pathology.

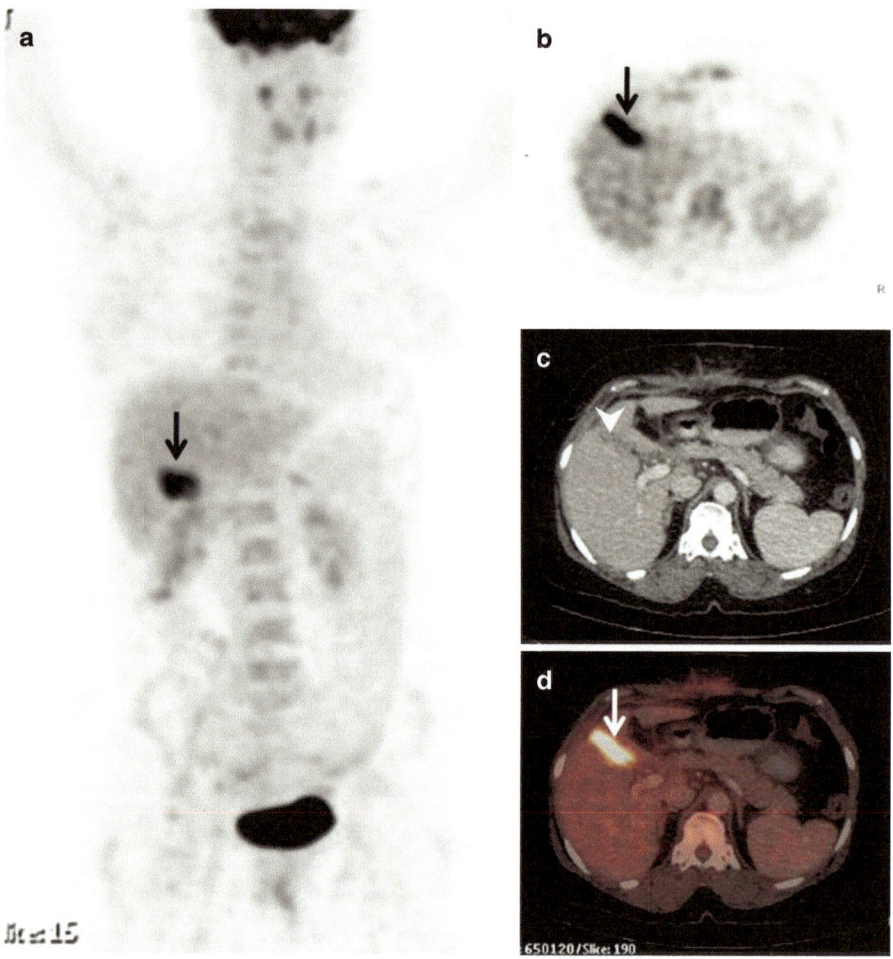

Fig. 5.6 False-positive PET/CT after recent cholecystectomy. Coronal MIP, axial PET and fusion PET/CT images show intense FDG uptake in the GB fossa (*arrows* in **a, b, d**) in a patient with recent history (4 weeks) of cholecystectomy for symptomatic gall stones. Persistent FDG uptake is due to postoperative inflammation and can be confused with residual disease. No obvious mass lesion is seen in the GB fossa on axial CT image (*arrowhead* in **c**)

Surgery in combination with chemo- and radiation therapy is used biliary and pancreatic cancers. Biliary drainage using percutaneous transhepatic technique (PTBD) or by endoscopic retrograde techniques (ERBD) is used to relieve obstructive jaundice before surgery or radiation and also as a palliative measure in advanced non-resectable tumours. Drainage tubes and stents cause inflammation of the biliary tree resulting in tracer uptake in the region of the stent [11] (Fig. 5.8). In most cases, uptake is along the stent and low grade in nature. Occasionally it can be intense and

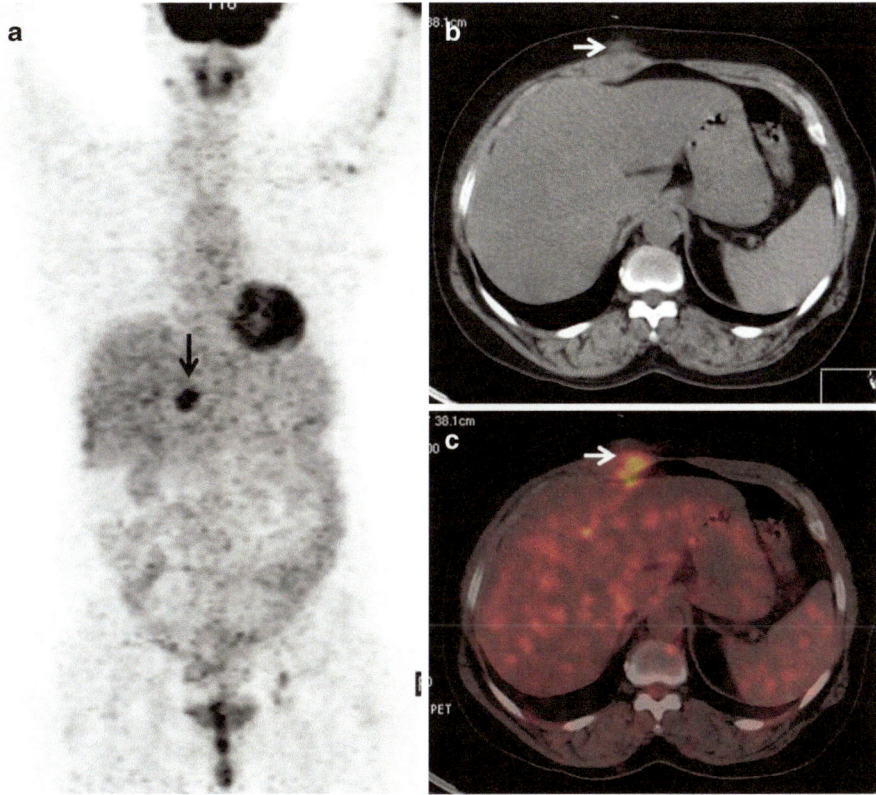

Fig. 5.7 False-positive PET/CT after laparoscopic cholecystectomy. Coronal MIP and fused PET/CT images show focal FDG uptake in the anterior abdominal wall (*arrows* in **a**, **c**) corresponding to the ill-defined soft tissue at the laparoscopic port site. Biopsy revealed inflammation. This finding can simulate port site metastasis

may mimic malignant disease. Intense uptake along the stent can also mask underlying small malignant lesion. Cholangitis and cholangitic abscess are serious complications of biliary drainage tubes and stents and can impair quality of life (Fig. 5.9). Intense FDG uptake is seen in cholangitis and can closely resemble cholangiocarcinoma. Cholangitic abscesses can often be mistaken as metastatic disease. Distribution of FDG avidity in a linear branching pattern along the biliary radicles and a photopenic fluid-filled centre of an abscess are important imaging features that can help differentiate inflammation from malignancy. Pancreatitis is also seen as a complication of biliary stenting as well as radiation therapy. Diffuse FDG uptake in the substance of the gland in combination with inflammatory CT features like pancreatic oedema, peripancreatic stranding and fluid collections can point towards the diagnosis of pancreatitis (Fig. 5.10).

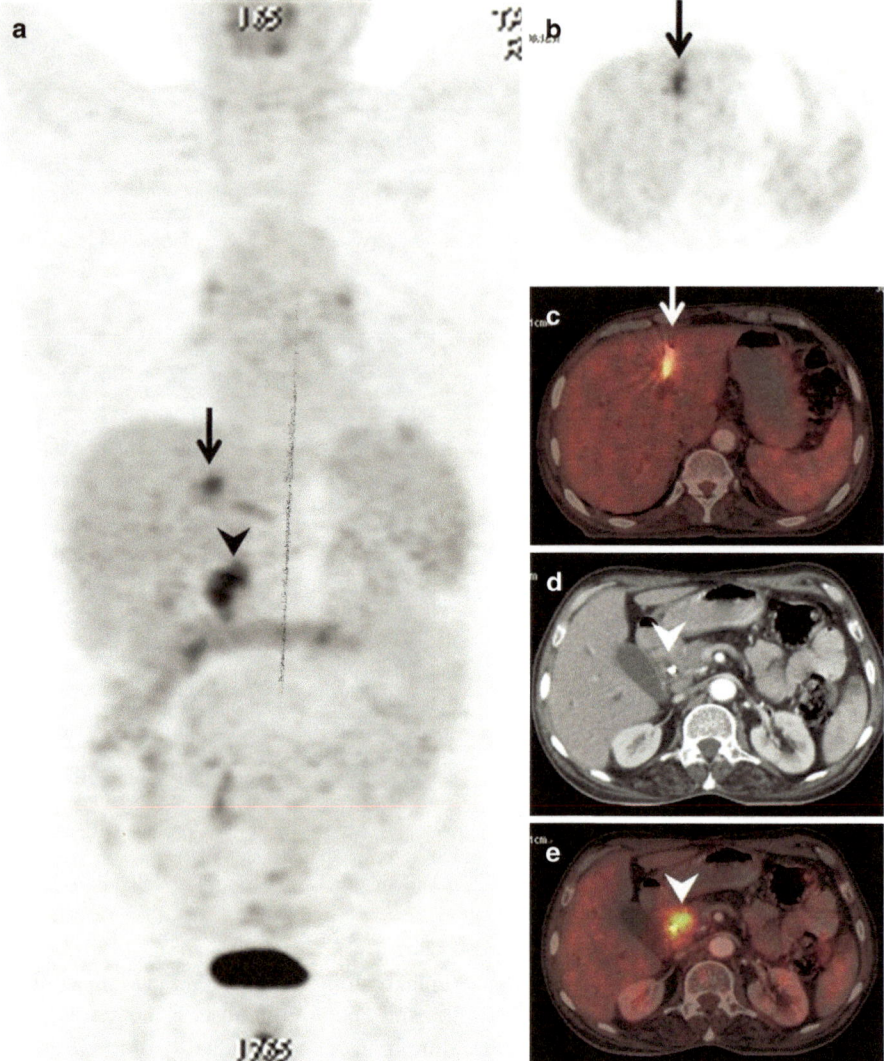

Fig. 5.8 False-positive PET/CT due to stent inflammation. Coronal MIP, axial PET images show focal uptake in the left lobe of the liver (*arrows* in **a, b**) corresponding to a percutaneous biliary drainage tube on fused PET/CT image (*arrow* in **c**). Coronal MIP and fusion PET/CT images show intense inflammatory uptake along the ERBD stent (*arrowheads* in **a, d, e**). Stent-associated inflammatory FDG uptake can be intense and mimic disease

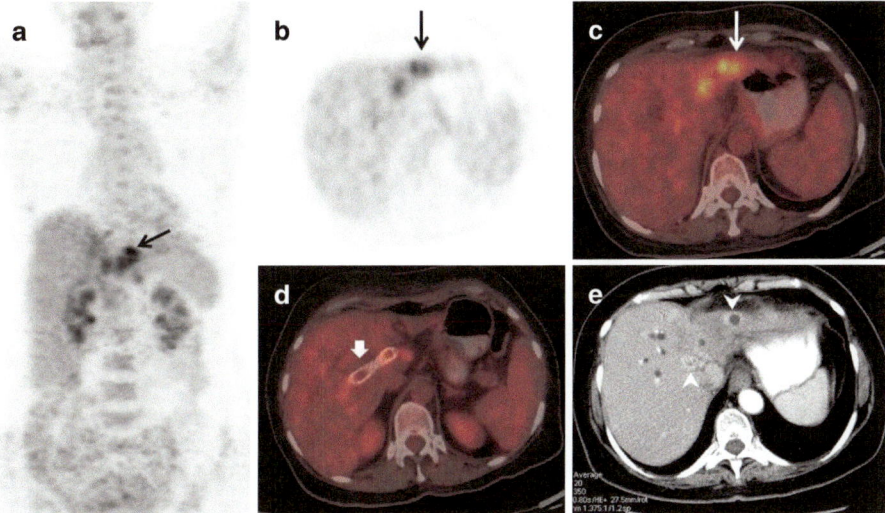

Fig. 5.9 False-positive PET/CT due to stent-related cholangitic abscess. Coronal MIP, axial PET and fused PET/CT show focal FDG uptake in the left lobe of the liver (*arrows* in **a**–**c**) corresponding to ring-enhancing abscesses seen on contrast CT (*arrowhead*). *Black arrow* seen in fusion PET/CT (**d**) show the ERBD stent

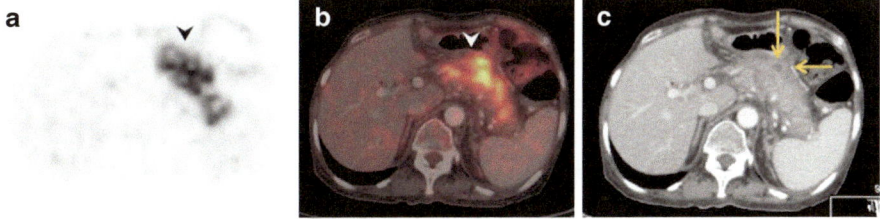

Fig. 5.10 False-positive PET/CT due to post radiation pancreatitis. Axial PET and fused PET/CT show intense FDG uptake in the body and tail of pancreas (*arrowheads* in **a**, **b**). Oedematous pancreas with peripancreatic fat stranding and small collections is seen on contrast CT scan which is diagnostic (*arrows* in **c**)

Conclusion

The anatomical and pathological complexity of pancreatico-biliary tumours leads to varying patterns of FDG PET appearances. Changes produced by surgery, radiation therapy and biliary drainage procedures and complications caused by them can lead to alterations in expected imaging appearances. Thorough knowledge of these imaging pitfalls is necessary to avoid errors in PET/CT interpretation.

Key Points

- The anatomical and pathological complexity of pancreatico-biliary tumours leads to varying patterns of FDG PET appearances.

- Cholangiocarcinoma can show variable FDG uptake depending upon the anatomic location, growth pattern and histological subtype.

- Lesions that are extrahepatic, infiltrative and mucinous in nature tend to show poor or no FDG concentration and can be difficult to localise on PET studies leading to false-negative results.

- FDG PET/CT has been found to be better in distinguishing MFP from pancreatic adenocarcinoma by virtue of lower tracer uptake in the inflammatory lesion. However, certain cases of MFP can show high FDG avidity due to the inflammatory process and can simulate malignancy.

- FDG PET can be falsely positive in cases of cholecystitis, and differentiation from malignancy can be difficult.

- Patients after laparoscopic cholecystectomy for unsuspected gall bladder cancer occasionally develop metastasis at the site of laparoscopy ports. PET/CT can detect port site metastases by demonstrating increased FDG uptake in those regions.

- Persistent inflammation at the port site causes FDG avidity that can mimic a metastatic deposit.

- Intense FDG uptake is seen in cholangitis and can closely resemble cholangiocarcinoma.

- Distribution of the FDG avidity in a linear branching pattern along the biliary radicles and a photopenic fluid-filled centre of an abscess are important imaging features that can help differentiate inflammation from malignancy.

- Diffuse FDG uptake in the substance of the gland in combination with inflammatory CT features like pancreatic oedema, peripancreatic stranding and fluid collections can point towards the diagnosis of pancreatitis.

References

1. Kato T, Tsukamoto E, Kuge Y, Katoh C, Nambu T, Nobuta A, et al. Clinical role of [18] F-FDG PET for initial staging of patients with extrahepatic bile duct cancer. Eur J Nucl Med. 2002;29:1047e54.
2. Anderson CD, Rice MH, Pinson CW, Chapman WC, Chari RS, Delbeke D. Fluorodeoxyglucose PET imaging in the evaluation of gallbladder carcinoma and cholangiocarcinoma. J Gastrointest Surg. 2004;8:90e7.
3. Fritscher-Ravens A, Bohuslavizki KH, Broering DC, Jenicke L, Schafer H, Buchert R, et al. FDG PET in the diagnosis of hilar cholangiocarcinoma. Nucl Med Commun. 2001;22:1277e85.

4. Pedrazzoli S, Sperti C, Pasquali C, Bissoli S, Chierichetti F. Comparison of international con-sensus guidelines versus 18-FDG PET in detecting malignancy of intraductal papillary muci-nous neoplasms of the pancreas. Ann Surg. 2011;254(6):971.
5. Schick V, Franzius C, Beyna T, et al. Diagnostic impact of 18F-FDG PET-CT evaluating solid pancreatic lesions versus endosonography, endoscopic retrograde cholangio-pancreatography with intraductal ultrasonography and abdominal ultrasound. Eur J Nucl Med Mol Imaging. 2008;35:1775–85.
6. van Kouwen MC, Jansen JB, van Goor H, de Castro S, Oyen WJ, Drenth JP. FDG-PET is able to detect pancreatic carcinoma in chronic pancreatitis. Eur J Nucl Med Mol Imaging. 2005;32:399–404.
7. Koh T, Taniguchi H, Yamaguchi A, Kunishima S, Yamagishi H. Diffcerential diagnosis of gallbladder cancer using positron emission tomography with fluorine-18-labeled fluoro-deoxyglucose (FDG-PET). J Surg Oncol. 2003;84:74–81.
8. Oe A, Kawabe J, Torii K, Kawamura E, Higashiyama S, Kotani J, et al. Distinguishing benign from malignant gallbladder wall thickening using FDG-PET. Ann Nucl Med. 2006;20:699–703.
9. Abouzied MM, Crawford ES, Nabi HA. 18F-FDG imaging: pitfalls and artifacts. J Nucl Med Technol. 2005;33:145–55.
10. JB H, Sun XN, Xu J, He C. Port site and distant metastases of gallbladder cancer after laparo-scopic cholecystectomy diagnosed by positron emission tomography. World J Gastroenterol. 2008;14:6428–31.
11. Corvera CU, Blumgart LH, Akhurst T, DeMatteo RP, D'Angelica M, Fong Y, Jarnagin WR. 18F-fluorodeoxyglucose positron emission tomography influences management decisions in patients with biliary cancer. J Am Coll Surg. 2008;206:57–65.

Hepatic Malignancies and FDG PET/CT

6

Sneha Shah, Nilendu Purandare, Ameya Puranik,
Archi Agrawal, and Venkatesh Rangarajan

Contents

Malignancies of the liver can be primary which include hepatocellular cancers (HCC) predominantly in adults and hepatoblastomas seen in children or secondaries—commonest from colorectal primary.

This article shall discuss the utility of FDG PET/CT in management of primary hepatic tumors and metastatic disease from colorectal malignancies.

6.1 Hepatocellular Carcinoma

Hepatocellular carcinoma is a disease which frequently occurs in the patients with chronic liver disease – secondary to injury caused by either hepatitis or alcoholic intake.

S. Shah (✉) • N. Purandare • A. Puranik • A. Agrawal • V. Rangarajan
Department of Nuclear Medicine and Molecular Imaging, Tata Memorial Centre,
Mumbai, Maharashtra, India
e-mail: snehahv@gmail.com

© Springer International Publishing AG 2018   53
N. Purandare, S. Shah (eds.), *PET/CT in Hepatobiliary and Pancreatic
Malignancies*, Clinicians' Guides to Radionuclide Hybrid Imaging,
DOI 10.1007/978-3-319-60507-4_6

6.1.1 Staging

The outcome of these tumors depends on the stage of the disease at presentation; larger tumors and metastatic disease have poorer outcomes. Staging of HCC is generally done using a triple-phase contrast-enhanced computed tomography (CT) scan or magnetic resonance imaging (MRI) of the abdominal region for local evaluation, and metastatic work-up includes bone scan and a CT chest.

Fluorodeoxyglucose positron emission tomography/computed tomography (FDG PET/CT) extrapolates the Warburg effect, increasing glucose utilization by malignant tissue which is identified by overexpression of GLUT receptor on tumor sites. However, HCC cells show varied glucose receptor expression and hence the uptake of fluorodeoxyglucose (FDG) is variable [1–3].

The sensitivity of FDG PET or PET/CT for identifying primary HCC ranges from 50 to 65% as seen in various studies [2, 4, 5] (Figs. 6.1 and 6.2).

HCC with metastases have a poor prognosis with limited treatment options, while locally advanced HCC in the absence of extrahepatic spread could be offered aggressive local therapies; thus, accurate staging helps triage patients. FDG PET has been useful in the detection of distant metastases of HCC and fares better than conventional imaging modalities for detection of bony involvement while showing similar detection rates for lung and nodal disease [6, 7] (Fig. 6.3).

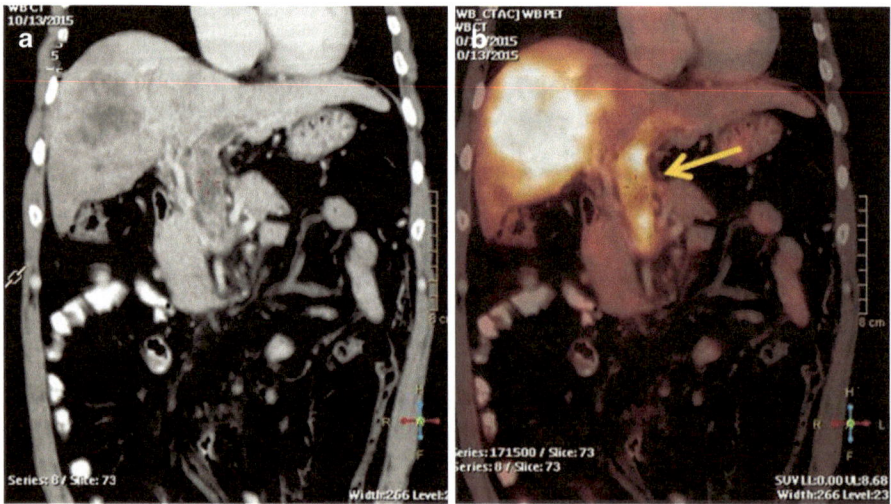

Fig. 6.1 Patient with HCC involving the right lobe of the liver as seen by the irregular hypodense lesion on the coronal section of CECT images (**a**) involving seg IV/VIII/VII and V and presence of right portal vein (PV) thrombosis, extending to MPV and SMV. FDG PET/CT done for staging shows intense FDG uptake in the primary mass (**b**) involving the lesion in right lobe of the liver with linear uptake (*arrow*) correlating with the tumor thrombus in the portal vein

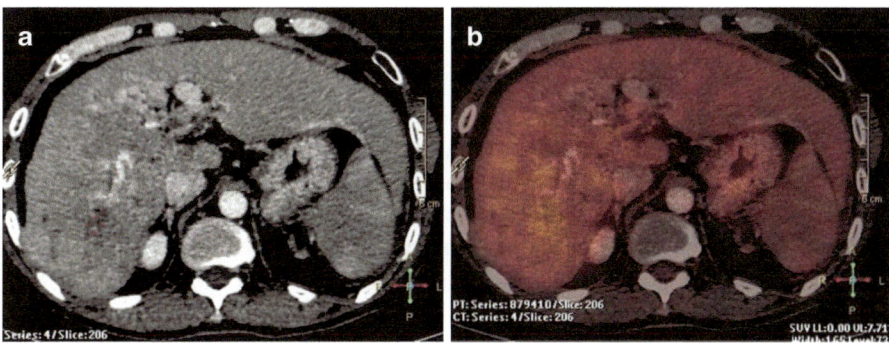

Fig. 6.2 12 × 9 × 9 cm mass in the right lobe of the liver with thrombosis of the right and main portal vein as seen on the transaxial CECT images (**a**). The correlative transaxial images of the FDG PET/CT study show no significant FDG uptake in the liver lesion (**b**) suggestive of a tumor with good biology

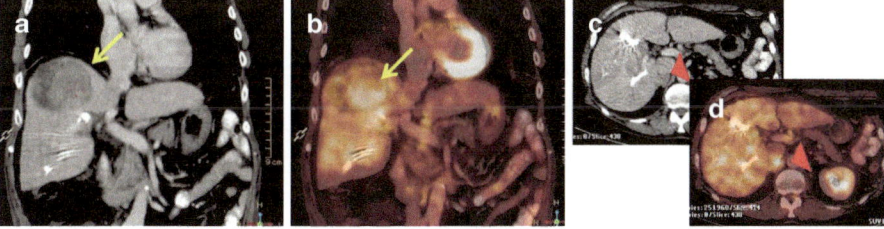

Fig. 6.3 A case of intermediate HCC involving the right lobe of the liver treated with TACE and planned for TARE. FDG PET/CT images show FDG uptake in the residual disease within the large heterogeneous lesion in the right lobe of the liver (*arrow* in **a, b**). Also noted is the FDG uptake in the metastatic nodule in the right adrenal gland on the transaxial and coronal-fused PET/CT images (*arrow head* in **c, d**)

A systemic review and meta-analysis evaluating FDG PET or PET/CT in extra-hepatic metastases and recurrent disease included eight studies and showed pooled estimates of sensitivity, specificity, positive likelihood ratio, and negative likelihood ratio of FDG PET (PET/CT) in the detection of extrahepatic metastases at 76.6% (95% CI, 68.7–83.3%), 98.0% (95% CI, 92.8–99.8%), 14.68 (95% CI, 5.5–39.14), and 0.28 (95% CI, 0.20–0.40), respectively [8].

Few studies which tried to evaluate its role as a biologic marker identified that tumors with a higher density of glucose receptors tend to be aggressive; hence, tumors which show greater FDG uptake could represent a disease with a bad biology [3, 9].

Tumors with no FDG uptake have better outcomes [10], while among FDG-avid tumors, those with higher FDG uptake show poor outcomes as compared with tumors with lower FDG concentrations. Tumors with a greater FDG concentration also tend to show a shorter doubling time and present with higher stage of disease [11–13].

6.1.2 Treatment Response Assessment

Local targeted treatment (LRT) for HCC exploits the pathophysiology of dual blood supply of hepatic tumors. It blocks the predominant arterial blood supply leading to reduction in blood flow and cell death via either ischemia, thermal/coagulation, or radiation effect which do not result in tumor shrinkage [14, 15], but show necrosis and reduction in the enhancement pattern which are not accounted in RECIST 1 or RECIST 1.1 criteria. The newer guidelines have incorporated the enhancement criteria (mRECIST) and necrotic parameters in the response assessment of HCC [16–18].

Identifying enhancement features could be difficult due to benign posttreatment inflammatory changes, or a heterogeneous nature of the tumor environment and functional imaging like diffusion-weighted magnetic resonance (DWMRI) or FDG PET/CT is recommended.

Response assessment with FDG PET/CT is done either by visual assessment of the tumor site in the pre- and post-therapy scans in comparison with blood pool uptakes or by calculating the reduction of FDG uptake at the tumor site using various semiquantitative or quantitative methods, e.g., ratio of tumor SUV to the liver or mediastinum or SUV max. Studies show better survival and event-free rates in patients who depict significant reduction in the uptakes at the tumor site [19, 20]. When compared to conventional imaging methods like CECT, FDG PET/CT showed a higher sensitivity in identifying residual viable tissue which is generally seen as a focal eccentric uptake in the periphery [21, 22] (Fig. 6.4).

In a bid to standardize the response assessment of solid tumors using FDG PET/CT, the PERCIST criteria was suggested by Wahl et al., which is adapted from the anatomical-based RECIST 1.1 principle and measures the FDG standard uptake (lean) in up to five index lesions (up to two lesions per organ) with highest FDG uptake. The response is expressed as percentage change in peak standard uptake of sum of lesions of baseline and posttreatment scans [23] (Table 6.1).

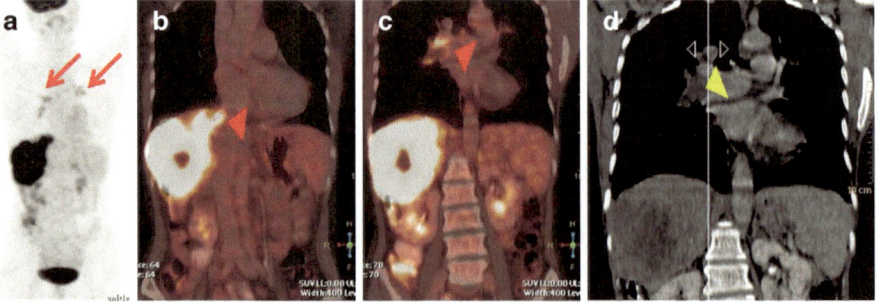

Fig. 6.4 Case of HCC involving the right lobe of the liver with portal thrombosis, patient was planned for trans arterial radioembolization and hence referred for a staging FDG PET/CT study. Intense FDG uptake was seen in the tumor involving a large part of the right lobe with uptake also seen in the portal vein thrombosis as seen on the MIP (**a**) and the coronal fused images (*arrow head* in **b**). Increased uptake is seen in the thoracic region bilaterally on the MIP image (*arrows* in **a**) which corresponds to filling defect seen in the pulmonary vein in the coronal-fused images (*arrow head* in **c**). The CECT of the thoracic region in the coronal image confirms the presence of bilateral pulmonary thrombosis (*arrow head* in **d**)

Table 6.1 Criterias for assessment of treatment response to conventional and targeted therapies (adapted from [24])

	RECIST 1.1	WHO	EASL	mRECIST	PERCIST
Complete response (CR)	Disappearance of all TL (up to 2 liver lesions)	Disappearance of all TL	Disappearance of all VL	Disappearance of all VL (up to 2 measurable liver lesions)	Disappearance of FDG uptake in the target lesions
Partial response (PR)	≥30% reduction in sum of greatest dimensional diameter of TL (compared to the baseline sum of diameter of TL)	≥50% reduction in the sum of products of bidimensional diameter of TL (as compared to the baseline sum of diameters)	≥50% reduction in the sum of products of bidimensional diameter of VL (as compared to the baseline sum of diameters)	≥30% reduction in sum of greatest dimensional diameter of VL (compared to the baseline sum of diameters)	Minimum reduction of 30% of SUV (lean) in measurable target lesion
Progressive disease (PD)	≥20% increase in the sum of diameter of TL (compared to the smallest sum of diameter of TL recorded since treatment started)	≥25% increase in the sum of diameter of TL (compared to the smallest sum of diameter of TL recorded since treatment started)	≥25% increase in the sum of diameter of VL (compared to the smallest sum of diameter of VL recorded since treatment started)	≥20% increase in the sum of diameter of VL (compared to the smallest sum of diameter of VL recorded since treatment started)	Increase of >30% of SUV (lean) or a new lesion identified on
Stable disease	Any case that do not qualify for PR or PD	Any case that do not qualify for PR or PD	Any case that do not qualify for PR or PD	Any case that do not qualify for PR or PD	Any case that do not qualify for PMR or PMD

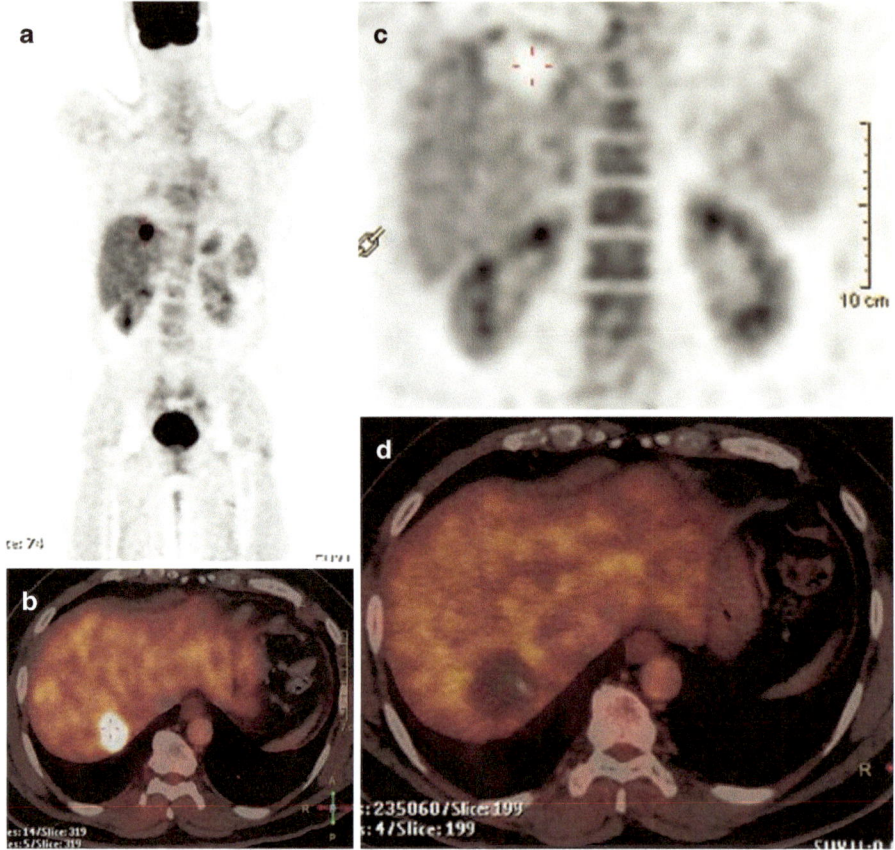

Fig. 6.5 Hepatic metastasis in a case of colon carcinoma, FDG PET/CT study done for restaging revealed a solitary liver lesion as seen in the whole body maximum intensity projection (MIP) (**a**) and well appreciated on the fused transaxial image (**b**). Post RFA FDG PET/CT study shows a photopenic area on the coronal PET image (**c**) which corresponds to the site of lesion with no uptake within or in the periphery as seen in the fused image (**d**) depicting completeness of the procedure

The ideal time to assess response would be at 3 months post therapy allowing for posttreatment-related changes to settle which could cause false-positive or equivocal readings.

Radiofrequency ablation is a localized treatment option for smaller tumors and those away from vessels. FDG PET/CT for this indication should be performed prior to initiation of inflammatory changes, i.e., within 6–12 h of procedure to avoid masking of the residual disease seen as a focal uptake in the periphery [25] (Fig. 6.5).

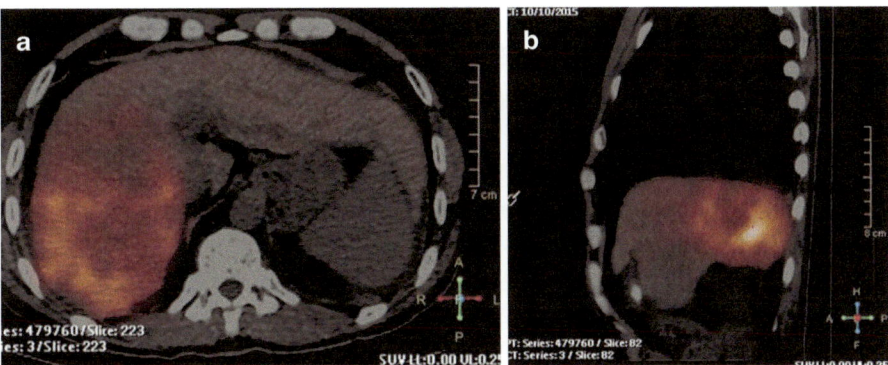

Fig. 6.6 Images acquired 3 h post 90 Yttrium therapy of patient in (**b**) reveal uptake at the primary tumor site in the right lobe—confirming delivery of the radiotracer into the hepatic lesion (**a**, transaxial and **b**, sagittal) and no tracer seen in rest of the liver parenchyma or elsewhere in abdomen—ruling out extravasation or leak of radiotracer

6.1.3   Utility of PET/CT in Evaluating Radioembolization of HCC

Post therapy scans in patients treated with 90 Yttrium tracers are evaluated with a bremsstrahlung imaging using the SPECT/CT scanner. Positron emissions from the Y90 radioisotope have been utilized to obtain an immediate post therapy PET/CT study. The advantage of this modality is the clear demarcation of region of radioisotope delivery and dosimetry to calculate actual dose delivered (Fig. 6.6). The presence of small extravasation of tracer into stomach or elsewhere is also identified which could have been missed on a pretreatment shunt evaluation dummy scan with colloids [26–28].

The posttreatment scan allows calculation of dose delivered to tumor which is a predictor of tumor response [29, 30] and to the normal liver which will help in identifying the dose leading to hepatic dysfunction.

6.1.4   Disease Recurrence

Early identification of local disease recurrence can be offered salvage treatment, and hence it is useful to identify extent of disease spread at restaging. FDG PET/CT has shown to be a helpful mechanism to identify sites of local or distant recurrence when a clinical suspicion is raised. FDG PET/CT showed an incremental value in patients with elevated tumor marker and negative imaging on CIMs and also better specificity and accuracy [31, 32] (Fig. 6.7).

A meta-analysis of eight studies discussed earlier showed a pooled estimate of sensitivity, specificity, and LR+ and LR− of FDG PET (PET/CT) in the detection of recurrent HCC to be 81.7% (95% CI, 71.6–89.4%), 88.9% (95% CI, 70.8–97.6%), 4.72 (95% CI, 2.21–10.07), and 0.19 (95% CI, 0.10–0.35), respectively [8].

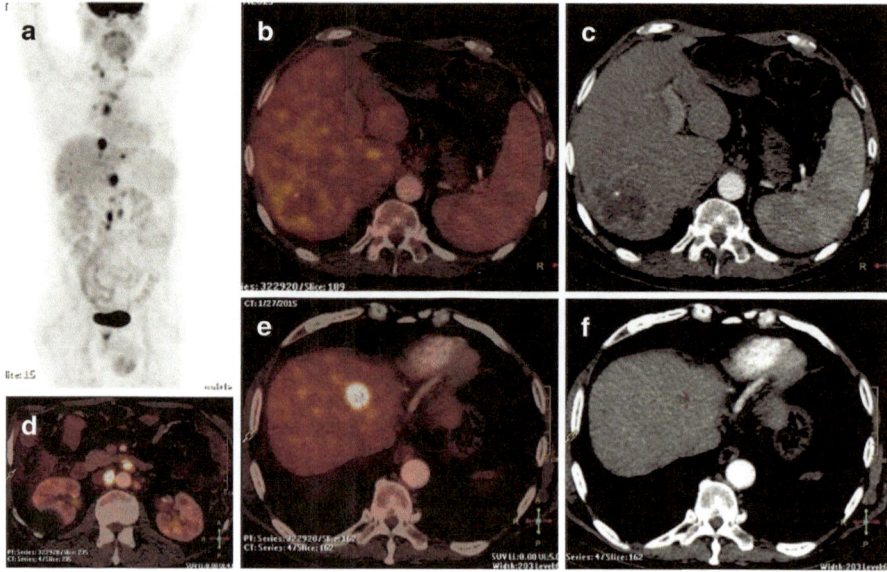

Fig. 6.7 Case of intermediate HCC treated with TACE had clinical suspicion of recurrence in view of elevated tumor marker. FDG PET/CT revealed absence of uptake in the primary site (**b**— CECT and **c**), focal FDG uptake seen in two lesions in the liver (**e**, **f**) and retroperitoneal nodes (**d**) and mediastinal and supraclavicular (**a**, *arrow*) metastatic nodal disease

6.2 Hepatoblastomas

Hepatoblastomas are glycogen-rich tumors and hence would have a high glucose receptor density leading to increased FDG uptake making it a suitable agent for staging these tumors; however, no significant literature is available pertaining to this [33]. Few studies which evaluated its role in restaging hepatoblastomas have found it to be a very specific test [34] and suggest an incremental value over conventional imaging (CT and MRI) in early recurrences [35] (Fig. 6.8).

Conclusion

Available literature suggests FDG PET/CT to be a prognostic factor while staging HCC and a good modality for assessing response to local therapies in intermediate HCC. There is not enough evidence to predict the role in hepatoblastomas.

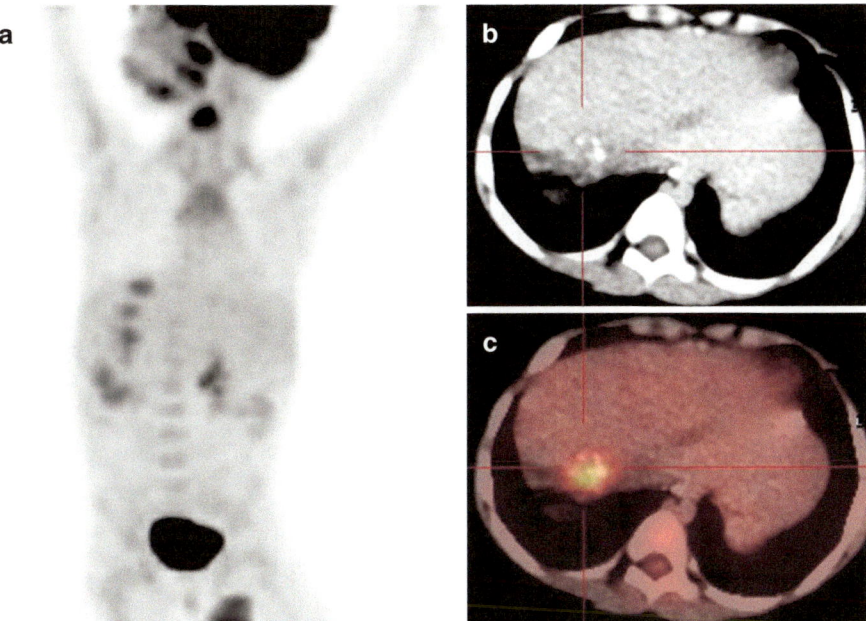

Fig. 6.8 Case of hepatoblastoma treated with chemotherapy followed by surgery and maintenance chemotherapy. On follow-up presented with elevated AFP level. Contrast CT scan did not reveal significant abnormality at the postoperative site or distant regions, a FDG PET/CT done revealed increased FDG uptake at the postoperative margins as seen on the MIP images (**a**) and on the fused transaxial PET/CT image (**c**) though no abnormality was seen on the correlative CT image (**b**). USG-guided biopsy confirmed recurrence on the diaphragmatic surface of the peritoneum overlying the liver

Key Points

- The sensitivity of FDG PET or PET/CT for identifying primary HCC ranges from 50 to 65% as seen in various studies.

- FDG PET has been useful in the detection of distant metastases of HCC.

- Tumors with no FDG uptake have better outcomes, while among FDG-avid tumors, those with higher FDG uptake show poor outcomes.

- FDG PET/CT showed a higher sensitivity in identifying residual viable tissue which is generally seen as a focal eccentric uptake in the periphery.

- The ideal time to assess response would be at 3 months post therapy allowing for posttreatment-related changes to settle which could cause false-positive or equivocal readings.

- FDG PET/CT is useful to identify sites of local or distant recurrence.

- FDG PET/CT showed an incremental value in patients with elevated tumor marker and negative imaging.

References

1. Lee JD, Yang WI, Park YN, et al. Different glucose uptake and glycolytic mechanisms between hepatocellular carcinoma and intrahepatic mass forming cholangiocarcinoma with increased (18) F-FDG uptake. J Nucl Med. 2005;46:1753–9.
2. Khan MA, Combs CS, Brunt EM, et al. Positron emission tomography scanning in the evaluation of hepatocellular carcinoma. J Hepatol. 2000;32:792–7.
3. Torizuka T, Tamaki N, Inokuma T, et al. In vivo assessment of glucose metabolism in hepatocellular carcinoma with FDG-PET. J Nucl Med. 1995;36:1811–7.
4. Ho CL, SC Y, Yeung DW. 11C-acetate PET imaging in hepatocellular carcinoma and other liver masses. J Nucl Med. 2003;44:213–21.
5. Wudel LJ Jr, Delbeke D, Morris D, et al. The role of [18F]fluorodeoxyglucose positron emission tomography imaging in the evaluation of hepatocellular carcinoma. Am Surg. 2003;69:117–24. discussion 124–126
6. Nagaoka S, Itano S, Ishibashi M, Torimura T, Baba K, Akiyoshi J, Kurogi J, Matsugaki S, Inoue K, Tajiri N, Takada A, Ando E, Kuromatsu R, Kaida H, Kurogi M, Koga H, Kumashiro R, Hayabuchi N, Kojiro M, Sata M. Value of fusing PET plus CT images in hepatocellular carcinoma and combined hepatocellular and cholangiocarcinoma patients with extrahepatic metastases: preliminary findings. Liver Int. 2006;26(7):781–8.
7. Kawaoka T, Aikata H, Takaki S, et al. FDG positron emission tomography/computed tomography for the detection of extrahepatic metastases from hepatocellular carcinoma. Hepatol Res. 2009;39:134–42.
8. Lin CY, Chen JH, Liang JA, Lin CC, Jeng LB, Kao CH. 18F-FDG PET or PET/CT for detecting extrahepatic metastases or recurrent hepatocellular carcinoma: a systematic review and meta-analysis. Eur J Radiol. 2012;81(9):2417–22.
9. Kwee TC, Basu S, Saboury B, et al. A new dimension of FDG-PET interpretation: assessment of tumor biology. Eur J Nucl Med Mol Imaging. 2011;38:1158–70.
10. Park JW, Kim JH, Kim SK, et al. A prospective evaluation of 18F-FDG and 11Cacetate PET/CT for detection of primary and metastatic hepatocellular carcinoma. J Nucl Med. 2008;49:1912–21.
11. Kong YH, Han CJ, Lee SD, et al. Positron emission tomography with fluorine-18-fluorodeoxyglucose is useful for predicting the prognosis of patients with hepatocellular carcinoma (in Korean). Korean J Hepatol. 2004;10:279–87.
12. Shiomi S, Nishiguchi S, Ishizu H, et al. Usefulness of positron emission tomography with fluorine-18-fluorodeoxyglucose for predicting outcome in patients with hepatocellular carcinoma. Am J Gastroenterol. 2001;96:1877–80.
13. Cho E, Jun CH, Kim BS, Son DJ, Choi WS, Choi SK. 18F-FDG PET CT as a prognostic factor in hepatocellular carcinoma. Turk J Gastroenterol. 2015;26(4):344–50.
14. Dhanasekaran R, Limaye A, Cabrera R. Hepatocellular carcinoma: Current trends in worldwide epidemiology, risk factors, diagnosis, and therapeutics. Hepat Med. 2012;4:19–37.
15. Arora A, Kumar A. Treatment response evaluation and follow-up in hepatocellular carcinoma. J Clin Exp Hepatol. 2014;4:S126–9.
16. Lencioni R, Llovet JM. Modified RECIST (mRECIST) assessment for hepatocellular carcinoma. Semin Liver Dis. 2010;30:52–60.
17. Bruix J, Sherman M, Llovet JM, et al. Clinical management of hepatocellular carcinoma. Conclusions of the Barcelona-2000 EASL conference. European Association for the Study of the Liver. J Hepatol. 2001;35:421–30.
18. Kallini JR, Miller FH, Gabr A, Salem R, Lewandowski RJ. Hepatic imaging following intraarterial embolotherapy. Abdom Radiol (NY). 2016;41(4):600–16. doi:10.1007/s00261–016–0639-5. Review. PubMed
19. Song MJ, Bae SH, Lee SW, Song DS, Kim HY, IeR Y, Choi JI, Lee YJ, Chun HJ, Lee HG, Choi JY, Yoon SK. 18F-fluorodeoxyglucose PET/CT predicts tumour progression after transarterial chemoembolization in hepatocellular carcinoma. Eur J Nucl Med Mol Imaging. 2013;40(6):865–73.

20. Ma W, Jia J, Wang S, et al. The Prognostic Value of ^{18}F-FDG PET/CT for Hepatocellular Carcinoma Treated with Transarterial Chemoembolization (TACE). Theranostics. 2014;4(7):736–44. doi:10.7150/thno.8725.

21. Kim HO, Kim JS, Shin YM, et al. Evaluation of metabolic characteristics and viability of lipiodolized hepatocellular carcinomas using 18F-FDG PET/CT. J Nucl Med. 2010;51:1849–56.

22. Song HJ, Cheng JY, SL H, et al. Value of 18F-FDG PET/CT in detecting viable tumour and predicting prognosis of hepatocellular carcinoma after TACE. Clin Radiol. 2014;70(2):128–37.

23. Wahl RL, Jacene H, Kasamon Y, Lodge MA. From RECIST to PERCIST: evolving considerations for PET response criteria in solid tumors. J Nucl Med. 2009;50(suppl 1):122S–50S.

24. Prajapati HJ, Spivey JR, Hanish SI, El-Rayes BF, Kauh JS, Chen Z, Kim HS. mRECIST and EASL responses at early time point by contrast-enhanced dynamic MRI predict survival in patients with unresectable hepatocellular carcinoma (HCC) treated by doxorubicin drug-eluting beads transarterial chemoembolization (DEB TACE). Ann Oncol. 2012;00:1–9.

25. Purandare NC, Rangarajan V, Shah SA, Sharma AR, Kulkarni SS, Kulkarni AV, Dua SG. Therapeutic response to radiofrequency ablation of neoplastic lesions: FDG PET/CT findings. Radiographics. 2011;31(1):201–13.

26. Elschot M, Vermolen BJ, Lam MGEH, et al. Quantitative comparison of PET and bremsstrahlung SPECT for imaging the in vivo yttrium-90 microsphere distribution after liver radioembolization. PLoS One. 2013;8(2):55742.

27. Zade AA, Rangarajan V, Purandare NC, et al. 90Y microsphere therapy: does 90Y PET/CT imaging obviate the need for 90Y bremsstrahlung SPECT/CT imaging? Nucl Med Commun. 2013;34:1090–6.

28. Wright C, Binzel K, Zhang J, Wuthrick E, Tung C-h, Knopp M. Post-radioembolization assessment of intrahepatic yttrium-90 microsphere biodistribution using next-generation digital PET/CT and comparison to current pre/post-radioembolization SPECT/CT methodologies. J Nucl Med. 2016;57(2):197.

29. D'Arienzo M, Chiaramida P, Chiacchiararelli L, et al. 90Y PET-based dosimetry after selective internal radiotherapy treatments. Nucl Med Commun. 2012;33:633–40.

30. Kao YH, Steinberg JD, Tay YS, et al. Post-radioembolization yttrium-90 PET/CT: part 2—dose-response and tumor predictive dosimetry for resin microspheres. EJNMMI Res. 2013;3:57.

31. Chen YK, Hsieh DS, Liao CS, et al. Utility of FDG-PET for investigating unexplained serum AFP elevation in patients with suspected hepatocellular carcinoma recurrence. Anticancer Res. 2005;25:4719–25.

32. Han AR, Gwak GY, Choi MS, et al. The clinical value of 18F-FDG PET/CT for investigating unexplained serum AFP elevation following interventional therapy for hepatocellular carcinoma. Hepatogastroenterology. 2009;56:1111–6.

33. Shiojiri N. Enzymo- and immunocytochemical analyses of the differentiation of liver cells in the prenatal mouse. J Embryol Exp Morphol. 1981;62:139–52.

34. Philip I, Shun A, McCowage G, Howman-Giles R. Positron emission tomography in recurrent hepatoblastoma. Pediatr Surg Int. 2005;21(5):341–5.

35. Cistaro A, Treglia G, Pagano M, et al. A comparison between ^{18}F-FDG PET/CT imaging and biological and radiological findings in restaging of hepatoblastoma patients. Biomed Res Int. 2013;2013:709037.

PET/CT in Pancreatic Malignancies

7

Ameya D. Puranik, Archi Agrawal, Sneha Shah,
Nilendu Purandare, and Venkatesh Rangarajan

Contents

7.1 Introduction

Pancreatic adenocarcinoma (PAC) accounts for about 85% of cases of pancreatic malignancies [1], and the term "pancreatic cancer" is sometimes used to refer only to that type. Imaging plays a central role in the management of this disease. Imaging facilitates establishing diagnosis, determining staging, monitoring treatment response, and detecting recurrence following surgery. Multiple modalities are involved, including computed tomography (CT), magnetic resonance imaging

A.D. Puranik (✉) • A. Agrawal • S. Shah • N. Purandare • V. Rangarajan
Department of Nuclear Medicine and Molecular Imaging, Tata Memorial Hospital,
Mumbai, Maharashtra, India
e-mail: ameya2812@gmail.com

© Springer International Publishing AG 2018
N. Purandare, S. Shah (eds.), *PET/CT in Hepatobiliary and Pancreatic Malignancies*, Clinicians' Guides to Radionuclide Hybrid Imaging,
DOI 10.1007/978-3-319-60507-4_7

(MRI), positron emission tomography with computed tomography (PET/CT), and endoscopic ultrasound (EUS). PET/CT combines functional information of PET with detailed anatomic information of multidetector CT [2]. Although the role of PET/CT in the diagnostic evaluation of patients with various abdominal malignancies is established, its role in pancreatic imaging is still evolving.

7.2   Imaging Modalities in Pancreatic Cancer

Abdominal ultrasonography is the first imaging modality for patients presenting with pancreaticobiliary symptoms or nonspecific abdominal pain. Diagnostic sensitivity of 90% has been reported by Karlson et al.; however, the retroperitoneal location of the pancreas obscured often by bowel gas, as well as the operator-dependent nature of the investigation precludes its use as an accurate diagnostic modality [3]. Multidetector CT (MDCT) is the modality of choice for diagnosis and staging of pancreatic cancers. PACs typically manifest as ill-defined hypoattenuating masses, with nearly 11% being isoattenuating on pancreatic and hepatic phase [4, 5]. MDCT has high sensitivity for detection of pancreatic cancers, ranging from 89 to 97%. Degree of vascular involvement and peritoneal and hepatic metastases on CT determine resectability of primary tumor [6]. MRI and MRCP are currently used as problem-solving tools for patients with PACs. There are specific situations where MRI is superior to CT: small tumors, hypertrophied pancreatic head, isoattenuating pancreatic cancer, and focal fatty infiltration of the parenchyma [7]. In small tumors, less than 3 cm, EUS is considered as an accurate modality for detecting these focal lesions; in addition, histological evidence can also be obtained by EUS-FNA [8, 9].

7.3   PET/CT in Pancreatic Cancer

7.3.1   Diagnosis and Staging

CECT is the modality of choice for diagnosis and staging; however, for tumors less than 2 cm, sensitivity significantly falls (approximately 83%). Moreover, tumors more than 2 cm in size and isoattenuating on CT account for almost 10% of PACs; these lesions are often missed on conventional CECT imaging [10]. Well-differentiated PACs are FDG-avid tumors, and hence metabolic imaging with FDG PET/CT picks up the primary site, while CT provides the morphological correlate. Okano et al. reported sensitivity of 100% and 40% for FDG PET and CT, respectively, for detecting lesions less than 2 cm [11]. As far as imaging pattern is concerned, focal FDG uptake is predictive of malignant etiology warranting further investigation [12]. Higher SUV (standardized uptake value) increases the sensitivity for depicting PACs, at the cost of specificity, as some of the infective and inflammatory lesions can sometimes show high SUV values. At the same time, ductal adenocarcinomas and mucinous/signet ring cell variants show low SUV values; a pattern typical for nonmalignant pancreatic lesions [13].

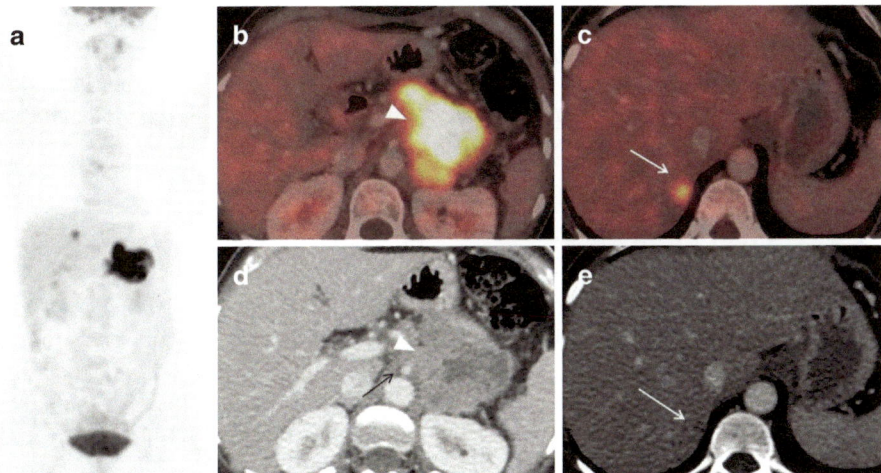

Fig. 7.1 FDG PET/CT in staging of pancreatic adenocarcinoma: MIP image (**a**) shows large area of tracer concentration in the mid-abdomen with focal tracer uptake in the liver. Axial PET/CT (**b**) shows FDG-avid large soft tissue mass in the body of pancreas with encasement of superior mesenteric artery on venous phase CT component (**c**-*arrow*) of PET/CT. There is intense desmoplastic reaction (**c**-*arrowhead*) with FDG uptake (**b**) delineating the actual tumor. Axial PET/CT (**d**-*arrow*) shows FDG-avid lesion in the liver which is seen as subtle hypodensity on CT (**e**-*arrow*) image suggestive of metastatic involvement

7.3.2 Local Staging

Pancreatic phase CECT (CT angiography phase) images of the aorta and the superior mesenteric artery (17–25 s after the start of contrast injection), pancreatic phase (35–50 s after the start of contrast injection), and portal venous phase images (55–70 s after the start of contrast injection), when acquired as a part of PET/CT protocol (Fig. 7.1b, c—arrow), provides best information about vascular involvement in terms of cross-sectional circumference, which determines operability [14].

PET, with its metabolic dimension, provides the actual site of disease, since PACs are often accompanied by a dense desmoplastic reaction (Fig. 7.1b, c—arrowheads). This, in addition, provides accurate site for biopsy and tissue sampling [15]. In actual clinical practice, most patients undergo triphasic CT for diagnosis and are further referred for PET/CT imaging in locally advanced or borderline respectable scenarios to rule out the liver and other sites of distant metastases.

7.3.3 Nodal Staging

Some studies reported modest improvement in the performance of FDG PET compared with CECT in patients with pancreatic masses, with sensitivity and specificity ranging from 30% to 49% and 63% to 93%, respectively, for evaluation of lymph nodes. Lesser tumor volume in affected lymph nodes and strong photon scatter from the primary tumor (penumbra effect) may partially explain the poor performance of FDG PET for lymph node staging [16, 17]. Metabolic information of FDG PET may complement that of CT for nodal staging, because even low-grade metabolic activity on fused imaging in a rounded centimeter-or-more-sized node may be indicative of nodal metastases.

7.4   Liver Metastases

FDG uptake in hepatic lesions strongly favors metastatic involvement; also the absence of FDG uptake in suspicious liver lesions seen on conventional imaging rules out metastases [18]. This dilemma arises mostly in case of solitary focal liver lesion that appears suspicious on triphasic CT/ultrasonography; here FDG uptake is a clincher as the presence of uptake favors malignancy (Fig. 7.1d, e, arrows) and further can be managed by liver-specific interventions.

In a study comparing the performance of hepatobiliary contrast-enhanced MR imaging and FDG PET, MR imaging was more accurate in depicting small liver metastases, with a reported accuracy of 97.1% compared with 85.3% for FDG PET [19].

7.5   Other Distant Metastases

Small volume disease in the form of nodular peritoneal implants often seen as stranding and rarely as frank "caking" pose a diagnostic challenge on CT, with reported sensitivity of 65–88% and specificity of 38–63% [20]. Peritoneal implants were found at staging laparoscopy in 7% of patients with locally unresectable pancreatic cancer and no evidence of metastasis at CECT [21].

Since PET/CT imaging is a whole body study, it is the best modality for detecting distant metastases at any site.

Most of the centers incorporate breath-hold plain CT of chest in PET/CT protocol, for detection of metastatic lung nodules. This is because detection of subcentimeter-sized nodules is beyond the resolution of even modern-day PET scanners, and hence plain thin-section breath-hold CT serves the purpose.

Thus, PET/CT impacts management change in patients deemed "operable" on conventional imaging, by detecting distant metastases, thus avoiding the cost of futile surgery.

7.6   PET/CT to Detect Disease Recurrence

PACs are naturally aggressive cancers, and following the natural history, after surgery, 72–92% of pancreatic adenocarcinomas recur locally within 2 years [22]. Locally recurrent tumors are usually not resectable; however, radiation therapy or

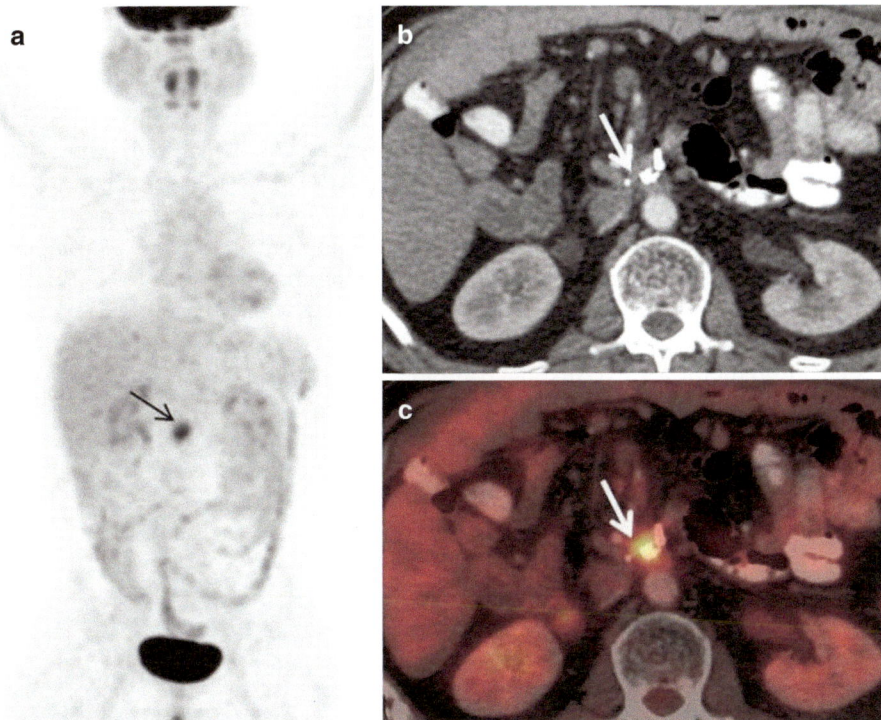

Fig. 7.2 FDG PET/CT for restaging. A 56-year-old female underwent Whipple's procedure for pancreatic adenocarcinoma involving body, followed by adjuvant chemotherapy; 6 months later, presented with rising CA19.9 levels, and hence was referred for PET/CT imaging. MIP image shows focal tracer uptake in the mid-abdomen (*arrow*), which corresponds to FDG-avid soft tissue (**b**-*arrow*) at the level of SMA origin (**c**-*arrow*) from abdominal aorta, thus representing local recurrence, with this being a typical pattern of local site recurrence

local ablation either with radiofrequency or cryoablation may be a palliative option. Postoperative changes in the surgical bed and early tumor recurrence have overlapping morphologic characteristics, as a result, differentiating between them is difficult on CECT. Moreover, it is often difficult to obtain an adequate tissue sample because desmoplastic reaction is known to be associated with pancreatic cancers. The use of FDG PET to depict tumor recurrence is promising, particularly when CT findings are equivocal [23, 24]. Increased FDG uptake in the surgical site at 3 months following surgery is usually indicative of recurrence (Fig. 7.2). The reported sensitivity of FDG PET for depicting tumor recurrence is 96% compared with 39% for CT and MR imaging [23]. Moreover, after resection, tumor relapse is depicted at FDG PET earlier than it is at CT, with higher sensitivity (98%) and specificity (90%) [24].

7.7   PET/CT to Detect Treat Response

PET combined with CECT plays a role in monitoring response to chemo- and radiation therapy in patients with unresectable pancreatic cancer [25, 26]. Significant reduction in FDG uptake may precede volumetric reduction at CT and may be proportional to the change in tumor size at subsequent follow-up examinations (Fig. 7.3). Therefore, earlier depiction of tumor response to therapy at FDG PET could influence the continuation or withdrawal of treatment [27]. Moreover, some recently published studies reported that FDG PET/CT might have prognostic value because tumors with a higher baseline SUV_{max} are more likely to recur in the early post-operative period. SUV_{max} is also an independent predictor for overall survival in patients with locally advanced pancreatic cancer [28, 29]. Postoperative inflammatory changes in the pancreas, radiation therapy, or stent placement may also cause some FDG uptake. To minimize these false-positive results, it is recommended that follow-up PET or PET/CT be performed at least 6 weeks after surgery [30].

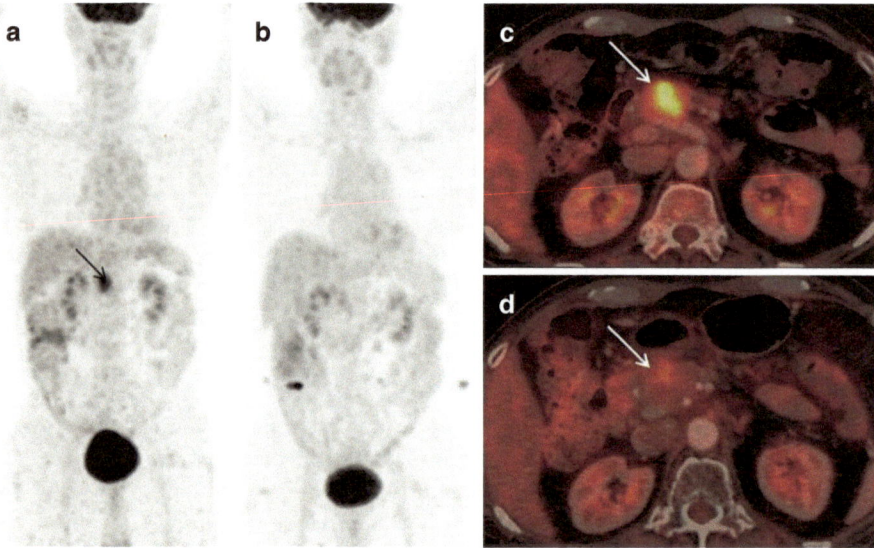

Fig. 7.3 FDG PET/CT in treatment response evaluation. A 46-year-old female patient presented with adenocarcinoma involving pancreatic head which was non-resectable received 6# chemotherapy; PET/CT study was performed to assess treatment response. MIP images (baseline-**a**, posttreatment-**b**) show regression in focal tracer uptake in mid-abdomen, which is seen as significant regression in size with near-complete metabolic regression at the primary pancreatic site (baseline, with no new lesions elsewhere, on axial PET/CT (**c**-baseline, **d**-posttreatment)

7.8 PET Tracers for Other Pancreatic Neoplasms

7.8.1 68Ga-DOTA-PET/CT

Neuroendocrine tumors represent 1–2% of all pancreatic neoplasms [31]; nonfunctioning tumors now account for 60–80% of such tumors [32]. Insulinoma and gastrinoma are the most common functioning islet cell tumors, accounting for about 32 and 9% of cases, respectively. Functioning tumors are detected earlier in their clinical course, when they are generally small in size.

As many as 90% of nonfunctioning tumors are malignant at the time of diagnosis, with more indolent biologic behavior than pancreatic adenocarcinoma [33]. Well-differentiated NETs, termed "carcinoids," often express somatostatin receptors (SSTR), whereas poorly differentiated variants express GLUT receptors making these tumors FDG avid. SSTR-specific radionuclides like Ga68-DOTA-TOC/NOC/TATE are the most sensitive radionuclides for this subset of tumors. Versari et al. [34] reported that 68Ga DOTA-TOC PET/CT has accuracy comparable to those of endoscopic US and multidetector CT for depicting primary neuroendocrine tumors in the duodenopancreatic area, with a sensitivity of 87% and specificity of 83%.

7.8.2 68Ga-DOTA-Exendin-4 PET/CT

The most common cause of endogenous hyperinsulinemic hypoglycemia in adults is an insulinoma. Endogenous hyperinsulinemic hypoglycemia is biochemically diagnosed by a prolonged supervised fasting test in an inpatient setting [35]. Small size of tumors is a limitation for localization by conventional imaging. Methods like intra-arterial calcium estimation and venous sampling are sensitive; however, their invasive nature poses risk of complications. Benign insulinomas have a high concentration of glucagon-like peptide-1 receptors (GLP R 1), which are good targets for in vivo imaging [36]. Early results with 68Ga-DOTA-exendin-4 PET/CT, which localizes to GLP-R-1, have shown good sensitivity for detection of these lesions [37].

7.8.3 18F–FDOPA PET/CT

The most frequent catecholamine-producing tumors are pheochromocytomas, which arise from chromaffin cells of the adrenal medulla (80–85%) or extra-adrenal paraganglia (15–20%). Imaging techniques are used to localize the primary tumor and to search for metastases. In case of pheochromocytomas, most tumors are benign, but 10–20% are malignant. The most specific agent which localizes to catecholamine precursor dopamine receptors is a F-18-labeled compound, fluoro-L-dihydroxyphenylalanine (F-DOPA) [38]. It has better resolution, imaging characteristics, and sensitivity than I-131 MIBG SPECT scintigraphy.

Key Points

- CECT is the modality of choice for diagnosis and staging.

- Well-differentiated PACs are FDG-avid tumors, and hence metabolic imaging with FDG PET/CT picks up the primary site, while CT provides the morphological correlate.

- For detection of lesions less than 2 cm, the sensitivity of FDG PET and CT is 100% and 40%, respectively.

- Ductal adenocarcinomas and mucinous/signet ring cell variants show low SUV values, a pattern typical for nonmalignant pancreatic lesions.

- In detecting nodal disease, there is modest improvement reported in the performance of FDG PET compared with CECT in patients with pancreatic masses.

- FDG uptake in hepatic lesions strongly favors metastatic involvement, but MR imaging is more accurate in depicting small liver metastases.

- The use of FDG PET to depict tumor recurrence is promising, particularly when CT findings are equivocal.

- Increased FDG uptake in the surgical site at 3 months following surgery is usually indicative of recurrence.

- The reported sensitivity of FDG PET for depicting tumor recurrence is 96% compared with 39% for CT and MR imaging.

- PET combined with CECT plays a role in monitoring response to chemo- and radiation therapy in patients with unresectable pancreatic cancer.

References

1. American Cancer Society. Cancer facts and figures. 2009. http://www.cancer.org/acs/groups/content/@nho/documents/document/500809webpdf.pdf. Last accessed 8 June 2012.
2. Kinney T. Evidence-based imaging of pancreatic malignancies. Surg Clin North Am. 2010;90:235–49.
3. Karlson BM, Ekbom A, Lindgren PG, Kallskog V, Rastad J. Abdominal US for diagnosis of pancreatic tumor: prospective cohort analysis. Radiology. 1999;213:107–11.
4. Bluemke DA, Cameron JL, Hruban RH, Pitt HA, Siegelman SS, Soyer P, et al. Potentially resectable pancreatic adenocarcinoma: spiral CT assessment with surgical and pathologic correlation. Radiology. 1995;197:381–5.
5. Brennan DD, Zamboni GA, Raptopoulos VD, Kruskal JB. Comprehensive preoperative assessment of pancreatic adenocarcinoma with 64-section volumetric CT. Radiographics. 2007;27:1653–66.
6. Bronstein YL, Loyer EM, Kaur H, Choi H, David C, DuBrow RA, et al. Detection of small pancreatic tumors with multiphasic helical CT. AJR Am J Roentgenol. 2004;182:619–23.

7. Hanninen EL, Pech M, Jonas S, Ricke J, Thelen A, Langrehr J, et al. Magnetic resonance imaging including magnetic resonance cholangiopancreatography for tumor localization and therapy planning in malignant hilar obstructions. Acta Radiol. 2005;46:462–70.

8. Cannon ME, Carpenter SL, Elta GH, Nostrant TT, Kochman ML, Ginsberg GG, et al. EUS compared with CT, magnetic resonance imaging, and angiography and the influence of biliary stenting on staging accuracy of ampullary neoplasms. Gastrointest Endosc. 1999;50:27–33.

9. Chen CH, Yang CC, Yeh YH, Chou DA, Nien CK. Reappraisal of endosonography of ampullary tumors: correlation with transabdominal sonography, CT, and MRI. J Clin Ultrasound. 2009;37:18–25.

10. Prokesch RW, Chow LC, Beaulieu CF, Bammer R, Jeffrey RB Jr. Isoattenuating pancreatic adenocarcinoma at multi-detector row CT: secondary signs. Radiology. 2002;224:764–8.

11. Okano K, Kakinoki K, Akarnoto S, et al. 18-F Fluorodeoxyglucose positron emission tomography in the diagnosis of small pancreatic cancer. World J Gastroenterol. 2011;17:231–5.

12. Soriano A, Castells A, Ayuso C, et al. Preoperative staging and tumor resectability assessment of pancreatic cancer: prospective study comparing endoscopic ultrasonography, helical computed tomography, magnetic resonance imaging, and angiography. Am J Gastroenterol. 2004;99:499–501.

13. Diedrichs CG, Steib L, Vogel J, et al. Values and limitations of 18-F-Fluoro deoxyglucose-positron emission tomography with preoperative evaluation of patients with pancreatic masses. Pancreas. 2000;20:109–16.

14. Zamboni GA, Kruskal JB, Vollmer CM, Baptista J, Callery MP, Raptopoulos VD. Pancreatic adenocarcinoma: value of multidetector CT angiography in preoperative evaluation. Radiology. 2007;245:770–8.

15. Mallery JS, Centeno BA, Hahn PF, Chang Y, Warshaw AI, Brugge WR. Pancreatic tissue sampling guided by EUS, CT/US and surgery: a comparison of sensitivity and specificity. Gastrointest Endosc. 2002;56:218–24.

16. Kauhanen SP, Komar G, Seppänen MP, et al. A prospective diagnostic accuracy study of 18F-fluorodeoxyglucose positron emission tomography/computed tomography, multidetector row computed tomography, and magnetic resonance imaging in primary diagnosis and staging of pancreatic cancer. Ann Surg. 2009;250(6):957–63.

17. Heinrich S, Goerres GW, Schäfer M, et al. Positron emission tomography/computed tomography influences on the management of resectable pancreatic cancer and its cost-effectiveness. Ann Surg. 2005;242(2):235–43.

18. Nakamoto Y, Higashi T, Sakahara H, et al. Contribution of PET in the detection of liver metastases from pancreatic tumours. Clin Radiol. 1999;54(4):248–52.

19. Sahani DV, Kalva SP, Fischman AJ, et al. Detection of liver metastases from adenocarcinoma of the colon and pancreas: comparison of mangafodipir trisodium-enhanced liver MRI and whole-body FDG PET. AJR Am J Roentgenol. 2005;185(1):239–46.

20. Tabuchi T, Itoh K, Ohshio G, et al. Tumor staging of pancreatic adenocarcinoma using early- and late-phase helical CT. AJR Am J Roentgenol. 1999;173(2):375–80.

21. Liu RC, Traverso LW. Diagnostic laparoscopy improves staging of pancreatic cancer deemed locally unresectable by computed tomography. Surg Endosc. 2005;19(5):638–42.

22. Sperti C, Pasquali C, Bissoli S, Chierichetti F, Liessi G, Pedrazzoli S. Tumor relapse after pancreatic cancer resection is detected earlier by 18-FDG PET than by CT. J Gastrointest Surg. 2010;14(1):131–40.

23. Casneuf V, Delrue L, Kelles A, et al. Is combined 18F-fluorodeoxyglucose-positron emission tomography/computed tomography superior to positron emission tomography or computed tomography alone for diagnosis, staging and restaging of pancreatic lesions? Acta Gastroenterol Belg. 2007;70(4):331–8.

24. Ruf J, Lopez Hänninen E, Oettle H, et al. Detection of recurrent pancreatic cancer: comparison of FDG-PET with CT/MRI. Pancreatology. 2005;5(2–3):266–72.

25. Kuwatani M, Kawakami H, Eto K, et al. Modalities for evaluating chemotherapeutic efficacy and survival time in patients with advanced pancreatic cancer: comparison between FDG-PET, CT, and serum tumor markers. Intern Med. 2009;48(11):867–75.

26. Bang S, Chung HW, Park SW, et al. The clinical usefulness of 18-fluorodeoxyglucose positron emission tomography in the differential diagnosis, staging, and response evaluation after concurrent chemoradiotherapy for pancreatic cancer. J Clin Gastroenterol. 2006;40(10):923–9.
27. Yoshioka M, Sato T, Furuya T, et al. Role of positron emission tomography with 2-deoxy-2-[18F]fluoro-d-glucose in evaluating the effects of arterial infusion chemotherapy and radiotherapy on pancreatic cancer. J Gastroenterol. 2004;39(1):50–5.
28. Schellenberg D, Quon A, Minn AY, et al. 18Fluorodeoxyglucose PET is prognostic of progression-free and overall survival in locally advanced pancreas cancer treated with stereotactic radiotherapy. Int J Radiat Oncol Biol Phys. 2010;77(5):1420–5.
29. Okamoto K, Koyama I, Miyazawa M, et al. Preoperative 18[F]-fluorodeoxyglucose positron emission tomography/computed tomography predicts early recurrence after pancreatic cancer resection. Int J Clin Oncol. 2011;16(1):39–44.
30. Blake MA, Singh A, Setty BN, et al. Pearls and pitfalls in interpretation of abdominal and pelvic PET-CT. Radiographics. 2006;26(5):1335–53.
31. Hruban RH, Klimstra DS, Pitman MB. AFIP atlas of tumor pathology: tumors of the pancreas—Series 4. Washington, DC: AFIP; 2007. p. 23–376.
32. Tan EH, Tan CH. Imaging of gastroenteropancreatic neuroendocrine tumors. World J Clin Oncol. 2011;2(1):28–43.
33. Rha SE, Jung SE, Lee KH, Ku YM, Byun JY, Lee JM. CT and MR imaging findings of endocrine tumor of the pancreas according to WHO classification. Eur J Radiol. 2007;62(3):371–7.
34. Versari A, Camellini L, Carlinfante G, et al. Ga-68 DOTATOC PET, endoscopic ultrasonography, and multidetector CT in the diagnosis of duodenopancreatic neuroendocrine tumors: a single-centre retrospective study. Clin Nucl Med. 2010;35(5):321–8.
35. de Herder WW, Niederle B, Scoazec J-Y, et al. Well-differentiated pancreatic tumor/carcinoma: insulinoma. Neuroendocrinology. 2006;84:183–8.
36. Christ E, Wild D, Forrer F, et al. Glucagon-like peptide-1 receptor imaging for localization of insulinomas. J Clin Endocrinol Metab. 2009;94:4398–405.
37. Antwi K, Fani M, Nicolas G, Rottenburger C, Heye T, Reubi JC, Gloor B, Christ E, Wild D. Localization of hidden Insulinomas with ^{68}Ga-DOTA-Exendin-4 PET/CT: a pilot study. J Nucl Med. 2015;56(7):1075–8.
38. Imperiale A, Sebag F, Vix M, Castinetti F, Kessler L, Moreau F, Bachellier P, Guillet B, Namer IJ, Mundler O, Taïeb D. 18F-FDOPA PET/CT imaging of insulinoma revisited. Eur J Nucl Med Mol Imaging. 2015;42(3):409–18.

PET/CT in Gall Bladder and Biliary Tract Malignancies

8

Archi Agrawal, Nilendu Purandare, Sneha Shah,
Ameya Puranik, and Venkatesh Rangarajan

Contents

In this chapter we shall discuss the role of positron emission tomography (PET/CT) in biliary tract malignancies—i.e., gall bladder cancer (GBC) and cholangiocarcinoma (CCA). Though carcinoma of ampulla of Vater could also be included here, it will be discussed separately in pancreatic malignancies.

8.1   Gall Bladder Cancer

Gall bladder cancer (GBC) is an aggressive and lethal malignancy and has a very poor outcome. It has a propensity to invade the hepatic parenchyma and the biliary tree resulting in high mortality rate with 5-year survival of less than 5%. It

A. Agrawal (✉) • N. Purandare • S. Shah • A. Puranik • V. Rangarajan
Tata Memorial Hospital, Mumbai, Maharashtra, India
e-mail: drarchi23@gmail.com

© Springer International Publishing AG 2018   75
N. Purandare, S. Shah (eds.), *PET/CT in Hepatobiliary and Pancreatic
Malignancies*, Clinicians' Guides to Radionuclide Hybrid Imaging,
DOI 10.1007/978-3-319-60507-4_8

metastasizes to the lymph nodes, causes peritoneal implants, and also spreads hematogenously. The diagnosis is often delayed due to nonspecific symptoms which are common to benign conditions like cholecystitis and cholelithiasis [1–3]. Most often GBC is discovered incidentally after surgical exploration for suspected benign gall bladder disease. It has been reported that approximately 1% of elective cholecystectomies harbor GBC [3]. More than 98% of GBC are of epithelial origin, and approximately more than 90% are adenocarcinomas. The commonest site within the GB is the fundus (approximately 60%), followed by the body (30%) and the neck (10%) [1].

8.2   Conventional Imaging Modalities for Diagnosis and Staging of Gall Bladder Cancer

Though ultrasonography (USG) is the first and commonest modality used for the detection of GB masses, CT definitely is a better modality for assessment of GB wall thickness and mucosal irregularities [1]. Contract-enhanced CT (CECT) also gives critical information regarding resectability of GB tumors, i.e., local, vascular and organ invasion, and the presence of lymph node metastases. But MRI is more accurate in differentiating benign from malignant GB masses. Magnetic resonance cholangiopancreatography (MRCP) and MR angiography help in diagnosing vascular and biliary invasion which are essential for deciding upon the resectability of GB tumors.

8.3   Role of FDG PET/CT in the Evaluation of Gall Bladder Malignancies

There is paucity of data regarding the use of ^{18}F–fluorodeoxyglucose (FDG) PET/CT in the evaluation of GBC. GBC concentrates FDG avidly and hence appears to have a potential role in staging [4]. FDG PET combined with diagnostic CECT helps in evaluation of the primary mass [Fig. 8.1], in evaluation of adjacent organ invasion (Fig. 8.2), and in detection of regional and metastatic nodal disease and peritoneal and distant metastases (Fig. 8.3). PET/CT is also helpful in demonstrating benign changes like cholangitis (Fig. 8.4), which are commonly seen coexisting with biliary tract malignancy. Ramos-Font et al., in a recent prospective study,

Fig. 8.2 ^{18}F–FDG PET/CT study of a 62-year-old lady showing hypermetabolic GB mass with loss of fat planes with the hepatic flexure of the colon (*arrow* in **a–c**) suggesting colonic infiltration

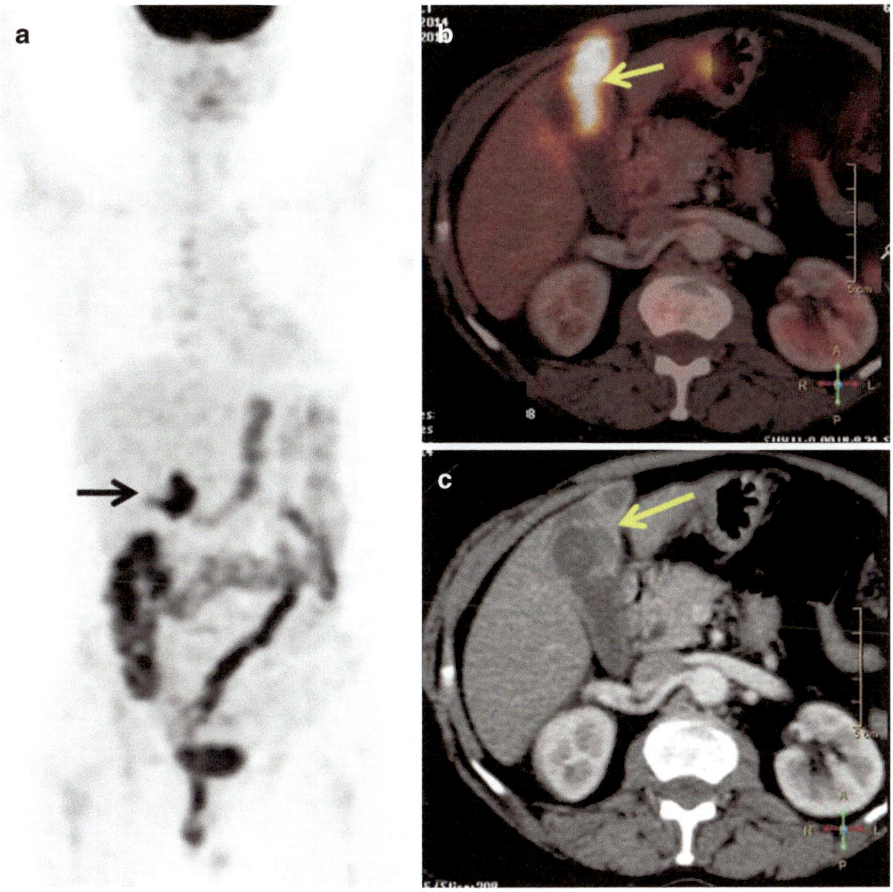

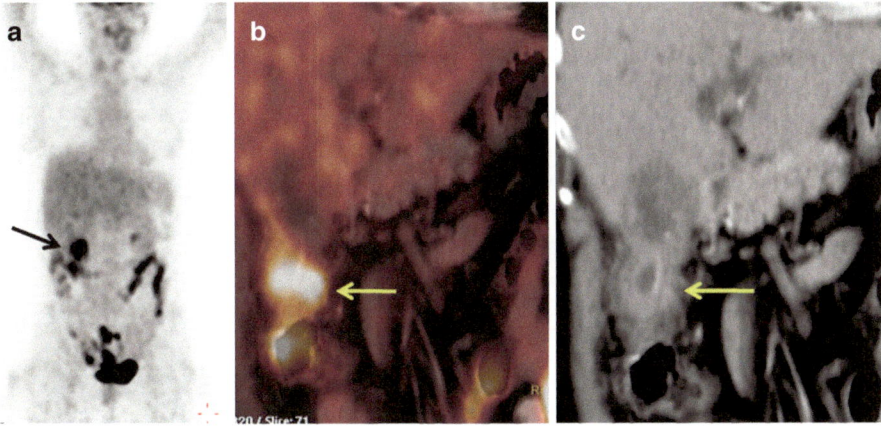

Fig. 8.1 51-year-old lady with suspected gall bladder cancer. ^{18}F–FDG PET/CT shows hypermetabolic mass with maxSUV 13.4 involving the fundus and body of the gall bladder (*arrow* in **a–c**). Histopathology post-radical cholecystectomy was adenocarcinoma of the GB

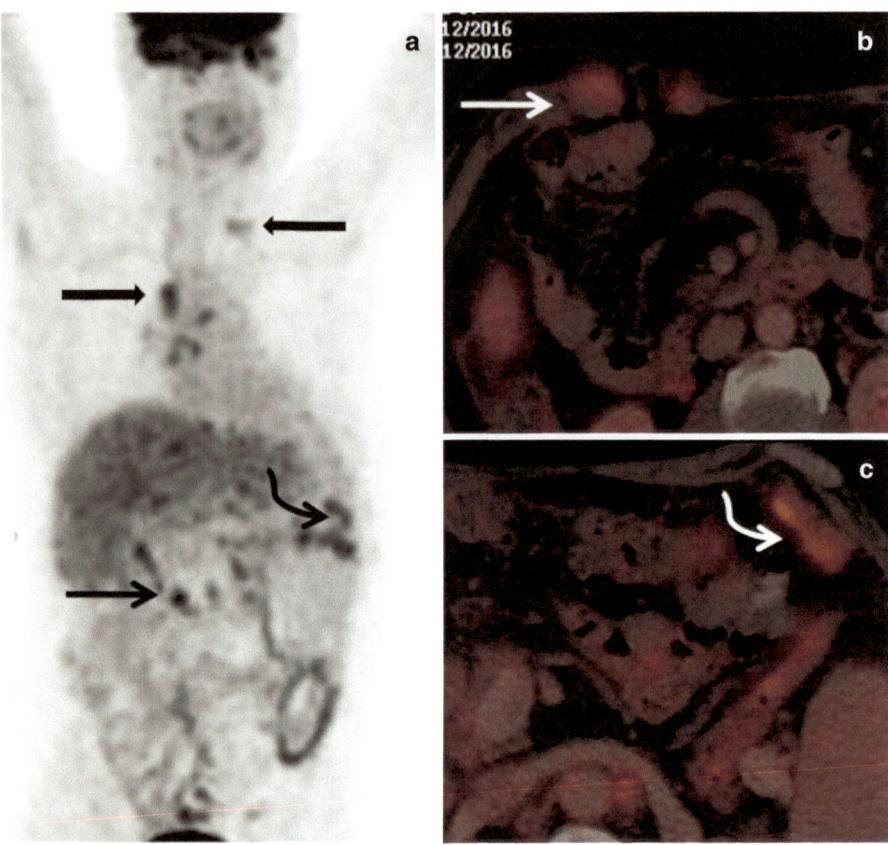

Fig. 8.3 55-year-old male, a case of GB carcinoma post-cholecystectomy. ^{18}F–FDG PET/CT shows hypermetabolic metastatic supraclavicular, mediastinal nodes (*block arrows* in **a**), anterior abdominal wall deposits (*arrow* in **a, b**), and peritoneal deposits (*curved arrow* in **a, c**)

showed an overall diagnostic accuracy of ^{18}F–FDG PET/CT, of 95.9% for the primary, 85.7% for lymph nodal metastases, and 95.9% for metastatic disease. In the restaging setting, the accuracy was 100%. FDG PET/CT led to change in management in 22.4% of patients [5]. In another study by Leung et al. done on 63 patients with incidental GBC postcholecystectomy, the sensitivity was 56% and specificity was 94%. It led to management change in 8% of patients [6]. PET/CT has also been used to stratify patients with incidentally detected GBC, to the most appropriate treatment depending on the presence or absence of distant metastatic disease [7]. A recent meta-analysis comprising of 13 studies demonstrated a sensitivity of 87% and specificity of 78% with area under curve (AUC) of 0.88 [8].

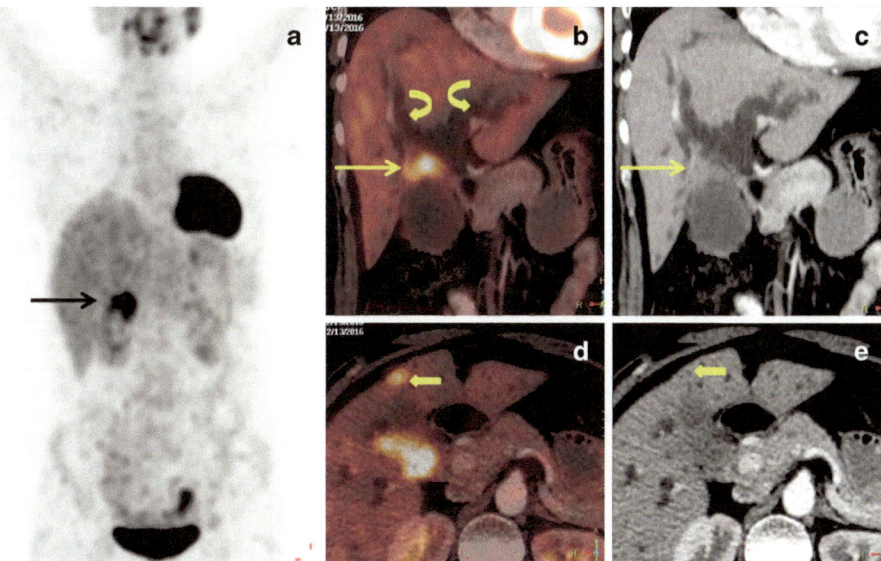

Fig. 8.4 ^{18}F–FDG PET/CT study of a 52-year-old lady with GB cancer. The study shows a hypermetabolic soft tissue mass (maxSUV 9.4) in the neck of the gall bladder (*arrow* in **a–c**) with bilateral intrahepatic biliary radical dilatation (*curved arrow* in **b**). The block arrow in **d**, **e** shows a focal hypermetabolic area in segment IVB, which was along the biliary radicals suggesting focal cholangitis (*block arrow*)

8.4   Role of FDG PET/CT in Prognostication

^{18}F–FDG PET/CT has a potential role in prognostication of patients with GBC. It has the ability to gauge the aggressiveness of a tumor based on increased glucose uptake in cancer cells. Hwang et al. demonstrated that maximum SUV (maxSUV) values were prognostic and were an independent predictor of overall survival (OS). They showed that patients with maxSUV <6 had longer survival as compared to patients with maxSUV >6. Also in multivariate analysis, patients with lower maxSUV in the pretreatment study and nonmetastatic disease survived longer [9]. Volume-based metabolic parameters like metabolic tumor volume (MTV) and total lesion glycolysis (TLG) are also prognostic in GBC. In a study by Yoo et al., TLG of the primary GB mass was an independent prognosticator for OS [10]. Also patients with positive FDG PET/CT have a shorter median survival as compared to those with a negative PET/CT study [11].

8.5   Cholangiocarcinoma

Cholangiocarcinomas (CCA) are rare adenocarcinomas (>90%) arising from intra-hepatic bile ducts, at the bifurcation of the hepatic ducts or from the distal common bile duct. The commonest form is that which arises from the bifurcation of the hepatic ducts (70%) and is called the Klatskin tumor. They are usually classified as intrahepatic or extrahepatic tumors. Intrahepatic can be further divided into mass forming, periductal, or intraductal based on the pattern of growth [12]. The patient usually is symptomless till an advanced stage is reached, and thus these are often diagnosed in late stage of the disease.

8.6   Role of Conventional Imaging Modalities

USG, CT, and MRI are the imaging modalities of choice for diagnosis and staging. These imaging modalities help in determining the size and extent of the tumor, biliary ductal dilatation, and involvement of regional lymph nodes [13–15]. Endoscopic retrograde cholangiopancreatography (ERCP) helps in obtaining brush cytology and biopsy.

8.7   Role of ^{18}F–FDG PET in Diagnosis of the Primary Lesion

^{18}F–FDG PET/CT has no advantage over these conventional imaging modalities in the diagnosis of CCA [16, 17]. The ability of PET/CT to detect a lesion depends on the location of the lesion. Studies have shown the highest sensitivity in the range of 91–95% and specificity ranging from 80 to 100% for intrahepatic bile duct lesions [18, 19]. This could be due to large tumor size of intrahepatic cholangio-carcinoma as compared to extrahepatic lesions. Another possibility is more accumulation of FDG in the malignant lesion as compared to the surrounding normal hepatocytes, where the turnover of ^{18}F–FDG is faster [20].

The ability of FDG PET to detect cholangiocarcinoma also depends upon the pattern of growth of the lesion—whether mass forming or infiltrative. The sensitivity for detection of a lesion is highest for mass-forming/nodular lesion as compared to periductal or infiltrating lesions [21, 23, 24]. In a study by Anderson et al., they found a sensitivity of 85% for nodular lesions and only 18% for infiltrative lesions [21]. Hilar CCA are well demonstrated on FDG PET/CT and also help in demonstrating intrahepatic biliary dilatation (Figs. 8.5 and 8.6).

In patients with benign inflammatory conditions like primary sclerosing cholangitis, abscesses, and granulomatous diseases, the results of FDG PET/CT should be reported cautiously; these conditions are potential mimics of cholangio-carcinoma. The ability of PET to detect CCA in patients with primary sclerosing cholangitis is debatable [20–22].

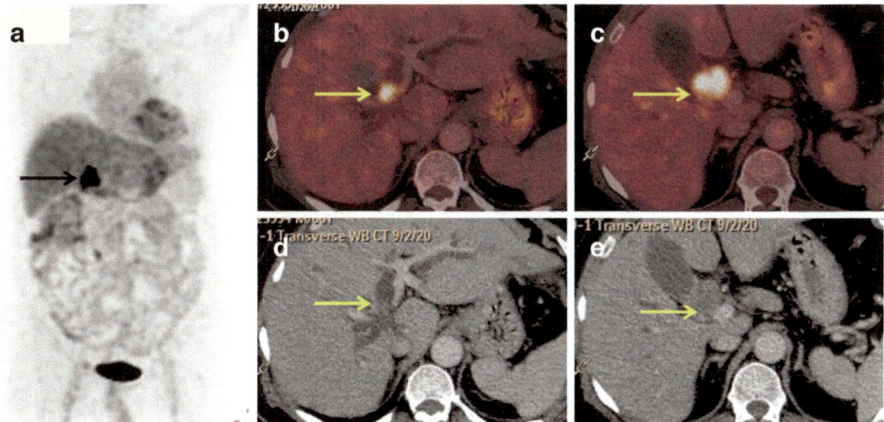

Fig. 8.5 ^{18}F–FDG PET/CT study of a 61-year-old male, diagnosed case of hilar cholangiocarcinoma. The study shows hypermetabolic mass at the confluence of right and left hepatic ducts (*arrow* in **a**–**e**) (maxSUV 13.51) with bilateral IHBR dilatation

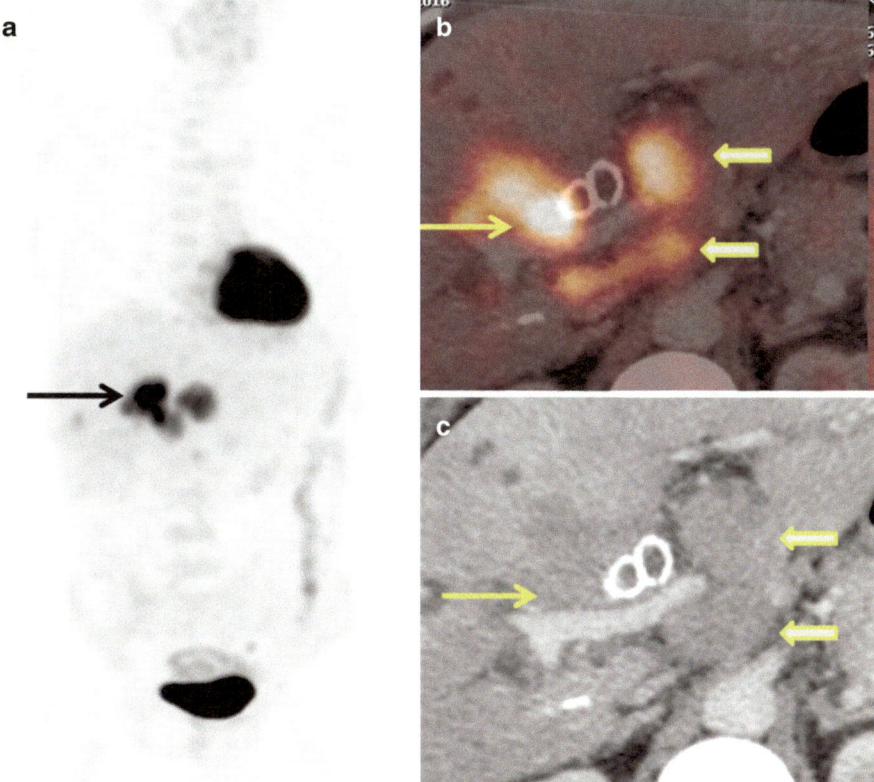

Fig. 8.6 ^{18}F–FDG PET/CT study of a male patient, 57 years, a case of cholangiocarcinoma. Hypermetabolic mass is seen at the hilar confluence (*arrow* **a**–**c**) (maxSUV 10.38) with multiple enlarged periportal lymph nodes (*block arrow*) (maxSUV 8.1)

8.8 Role of ^{18}F–FDG PET in Detection of Lymph Nodal Metastases

PET has a lower sensitivity (38–43%) and greater specificity (95–100%) in detection of involved nodes, as compared to CECT (SN 43–54%, SP 59–76%) [25, 26]. PET has an added advantage of detecting malignant nodes of less than 1 cm size, in contrast to conventional imaging, which is size dependent.

8.9 Role of ^{18}F–FDG PET in Detection of Distant Metastases

PET is highly accurate for the detection of suspected as well as unsuspected distant metastases. It has the ability to detect metastases not detected by conventional imaging modalities. It leads to change in management in up to 30% of patients by detection of distant metastatic lesions [21, 22].

The role of FDG PET/CT in the prediction of prognosis in CCA is not well established.

Key Points

Gall Bladder Cancer

- Gall bladder cancer concentrates FDG avidly and hence appears to have a potential role in staging.

- FDG PET combined with diagnostic CECT helps in evaluation of the primary mass, evaluation of adjacent organ invasion, and detection of regional and nodal and peritoneal and distant metastases.

- Diagnostic accuracy of ^{18}F–FDG PET/CT is 96% for the primary, 86% for lymph nodal metastases, and 96% for metastatic disease.

- ^{18}F–FDG PET/CT has a potential role in prognostication of patients with GBC.

- Maximum SUV (maxSUV) values are reported as an independent predictor of overall survival (OS). (Patients with maxSUV <6 had longer survival as compared to patients with maxSUV >6.)

- Patients with positive FDG PET/CT have a shorter median survival as compared to those with a negative PET/CT study.

Cholangiocarcinoma

- ^{18}F–FDG PET/CT has no advantage over conventional imaging modalities in diagnosis of CCA.

- In the detection of intrahepatic bile duct lesions, the sensitivity is in the range of 91–95% and specificity ranging from 80 to 100%.

- The ability of FDG PET to detect cholangiocarcinoma also depends upon the pattern of growth of the lesion—whether mass-forming or infiltrative.

- PET has a lower sensitivity (38–43%) and greater specificity (95–100%) in detection of involved nodes, as compared to CECT (SN 43–54%, SP 59–76%).

- PET is highly accurate for the detection of suspected as well as unsuspected distant metastases and leads to change in management in up to 30% of patients.

- The role of FDG PET/CT in the prediction of prognosis in CCA is not well established.

References

1. Levy AD, Murakata LA, Rohrmann CA Jr. Gallbladder carcinoma: radiologic-pathologic correlation. Radiographics 2001, 21:295–314.
2. Rodríguez-Fernández A, Gómez-Río M, Medina-Benítez A, Moral JV, Ramos-Font C, Ramia-Angel JM, Llamas-Elvira JM, Ferrón-Orihuela JA, Lardelli-Claret P. Application of modern imaging methods in diagnosis of gallbladder cancer. J Surg Oncol. 2006;93:650–64.
3. Duffy A, Capanu M, Abou-Alfa GK, Huitzil D, Jarnagin W, Fong Y, D'Angelica M, Dematteo RP, Blumgart LH, O'Reilly EM. Gallbladder cancer (GBC):10-year experience at Memorial Sloan-Kettering Cancer Centre (MSKCC). J Surg Oncol. 2008;98:485–9.
4. Agrawal A, Rangarajan V. Appropriateness criteria of FDG PET/CT in oncology. Indian J Radiol Imaging. 2015;25(2):88–101.
5. Ramos-Font C, Ramos-Font C, Gómez-Rio M, Rodríguez-Fernández A, et al. Ability of FDG-PET/CT in the detection of gallbladder cancer. J Surg Oncol. 2014;109(3):218–24.
6. Leung U, Pandit-Taskar N, Corvera CU, et al. Impact of pre-operative positron emission tomography in gallbladder cancer. HPB (Oxford). 2014;16:1023–30.
7. Goel M, Tamhankar A, Rangarajan V, Patkar S, Ramadwar M, Shrikhande SV. Role of PET CT scan in redefining treatment of incidental gall bladder carcinoma. J Surg Oncol. 2016;113(6):652–8.
8. Annunziata S, Pizzuto DA, Caldarella C, Galiandro F, Sadeghi R, Treglia G. Diagnostic accuracy of fluorine-18-fluorodeoxyglucose positron emission tomography in gallbladder cancer: a meta-analysis. World J Gastroenterol. 2015;21(40):11481–8.
9. Hwang JP, Lim I, Na II, et al. Prognostic value of maxSUV measured by fluorine-18 fluorodeoxyglucose positron emission tomography with computed tomography in patients with gallbladder cancer. Nucl Med Mol Imaging. 2014;48(2):114–20.
10. Yoo J, Choi JY, Lee KT, et al. Prognostic significance of volume-based metabolic parameters by (18)FFDG PET/CT in gallbladder carcinoma. Nucl Med Mol Imaging. 2012;46(3): 201–6.
11. Redondo F, Butte J, Lavados H, et al. 18F-FDG PET/CT performance and prognostic value in patients with incidental gallbladder carcinoma. J Nucl Med. 2012;53(515):515.
12. Blechacz BR, Gores GJ. Cholangiocarcinoma. Clin Liver Dis. 2008;12:131e50.
13. De Groen PC, Gores GJ, LaRusso NF, Gunderson LL, Nagorney DM. Biliary tract cancers. N Engl J Med. 1999;341:1368e78.

14. Gores GJ. Early detection and treatment of cholangiocarcinoma. Liver Transpl. 2000;6:S30e4.
15. Zech CJ, Shoenberg SO, Reiser M, Helmberger T. Cross-sectional imaging of biliary tumors: current clinical status and future developments. Eur Radiol. 2004;14:1174e87.
16. Kim JY, Kim MH, Lee TY, et al. Clinical role of 18F-FDG PET-CT in suspected and potentially operable cholangiocarcinoma: a prospective study compared with conventional imaging. Am J Gastroenterol. 2008;103:1145–51.
17. Petrowsky H, Wildbrett P, Husarik DB, et al. Impact of integrated positron emission tomography and computed tomography on staging and management of gallbladder cancer and cholangiocarcinoma. J Hepatol. 2006;45:43–50.
18. Moon CM, Bang S, Chung JB, Park SW, Song SY, Yun M, et al. Usefulness of 18F- fluorodeoxyglucose positron emission tomography in differential diagnosis and staging of cholangiocarcinomas. J Gastroenterol Hepatol. 2008;23:759e65.
19. Corvera CU, Blumgart LH, Akhurst T, DeMatteo RP, D'Angelica M, Fong Y, et al. 18F-fluorodeoxyglucose positron emission tomography influences management decisions in patients with biliary cancer. J Am Coll Surg. 2008;206:57e65.
20. Keiding S, Hansen SB, Rasmussen HH, Gee A, Kruse A, Roelsgaard K, et al. Detection of cholangiocarcinoma in primary sclerosing cholangitis by positron emission tomography. Hepatology. 1998;28:700e6.
21. Anderson CD, Rice MH, Pinson CW, Chapman WC, Chari RS, Delbeke D. Fluorodeoxyglucose PET imaging in the evaluation of gallbladder carcinoma and cholangiocarcinoma. J Gastrointest Surg. 2004;8:90–7.
22. Kluge R, Schmidt F, Caca K, Barthel H, Hesse S, Georgi P, et al. Positron emission tomography with [18F]fluoro-2-deoxy-D-glucose for diagnosis and staging of bile duct cancer. Hepatology. 2001;33:1029e35.
23. Nakeeb A, Pitt HA, Sohn TA, et al. Cholangiocarcinoma: a spectrum of intrahepatic, perihilar, and distal tumors. Ann Surg. 1996;224:463–473, discussion 473–475.
24. Jadvar H, Henderson RW, Conti PS. [F-18]Fluorodeoxyglucose positron emission tomography and positron emission tomography: computed tomography in recurrent and metastatic cholangiocarcinoma. J Comput Assist Tomogr. 2007;31:223–8.
25. Kato T, Tsukamoto E, Kuge Y, Katoh C, Nambu T, Nobuta A, et al. Clinical role of [18] F-FDG PET for initial staging of patients with extrahepatic bile duct cancer. Eur J Nucl Med. 2002;29:1047e54.
26. Seo S, Hatano E, Higashi T, Nakajima A, Nakamoto Y, Tada M, et al. Fluorine-18 fluorodeoxyglucose positron emission tomography predicts lymph node metastasis, P-glycoprotein expression, and recurrence after resection in mass forming intrahepatic cholangiocarcinoma. Surgery. 2008;143:769e77.

Index

© Springer International Publishing AG 2018
N. Purandare, S. Shah (eds.), *PET/CT in Hepatobiliary and Pancreatic
Malignancies*, Clinicians' Guides to Radionuclide Hybrid Imaging,
DOI 10.1007/978-3-319-60507-4